I AM A SICKLE CELL SURVIVOR

I AM A SICKLE CELL SURVIVOR
Ten Years and Still Counting

CAROL MARRIAM MULUMBA

© 2019 by Carol Marriam Mulumba

All rights reserved. No part of this book may be reproduced or transmitted in any form or by any means, electronic or mechanical, including photocopying, recording, or by any information storage and retrieval system, except in the case of brief quotations embodied in critical articles and reviews, without prior written permission of the writer.

Printed in the United States of America

ISBN Paperback: 978-0-578-60185-4

Book Design: Creative Publishing Book Design
Photos on pages 89-92 by White House Copyright 2010
Photo on cover page by Kristina Cilia, Copyright 2019

Table of Contents

Preface vii
Foreword. ix
Doomed Path 1
Texas. 5
Dr. Lockhart 9
Ford's Funeral 13
Hype. 17
Two-Month School Year 21
Central Line Surgery. 25
Just Like Home. 35
Hospital Anecdotes. 39
Blue Smiles 45
Drumroll Please: The Bone Marrow Transplant. 51
Indoor Trick-or-Treating 59
Temporary Solace 63
Home but Not Yet Free. 69
Baby Steps 73

Goodbye, My Second Skin 81
Hello, Mr. President. 87
Chore List. 95
Grandma Carol. 101
Alternative Path 107
Acknowledgments. 113
About the Author 115

Preface

I am a Sickle Cell Survivor, Ten Years and still Counting narrates the raw, straight-from-the-source story of an 18-year-old Sickle Cell survivor recounting her medical journey from frequent hospital visits, multiple absences from school, as well as an almost unconscious pull to be rid of what genetic shackles are holding her back. And all her memories were formed from the innocent cradle of her mind from when she was only a child. At seven years of age when she received the bone marrow and cord blood stem cell transplant. Carol's story before and now 10 years after the procedure is nothing short of an incredible make-over. The innocence but depth of this spell-binding narrative is more than just an eye-opener to the intricate challenges of sickle cell anemia. Her story renders a human face to sickle cell anemia and is the welcome handbook during an encounter with the debilitating and almost always, a fatal disease.

Foreword

I have often wondered about some of the experiences endured by my mother as a child with sickle cell. I can only pray that my mother was given the love and support that she needed during her journey with the disease. For me, the school year began like so many others with the Meet the Teacher session at Lackland Elementary School. Little did I know that I would get a first-hand glimpse into what a child diagnosed with sickle cell goes through or the pain of parents who love their child. As introductions were being made, I noticed a shy little girl who was not exploring the classroom like so many of her soon to be classmates. She was very well-mannered and stood very close to her mother who introduced the family and briefly began to share a history of Carol's condition. All I could hear was 'sickle cell' and my heart got set to help both academically and emotionally to ensure that Carol experienced the same first grade year as her peers. Many times during the year, Carol had to leave class to go to the nurse, be excused from activities in Physical Education class, or miss days from school. Her visits to the hospital with home tutoring on the weekends became a part of her routine. Even writing and trying to keep up with her classwork was a challenge. This is not acceptable as a routine for a six year old. She would share her big beautiful smile on the days that she felt well. Later in the year, she did a presentation about her condition to the class and her classmates understood.

Carol received her brother, Mark's bone marrow and cord blood stem cells during second grade. I visited her in the hospital when she was strong enough to receive visitors. We would read and watch videos together. I was so thankful that Carol was spared living the life that she experienced her first six years. I am extremely proud that she has accomplished much in eighteen years.

Throughout the years The Mulumba's and I have maintained a special relationship. Carol has many accomplishments already and will do great things in the future with her beautiful smile and courageous spirit. Carol, thank you for letting me be part of your journey.

Now, in her own words, Carol Mulumba can give you an insights into both sides; as a patient and as a survivor of sickle cell anemia.

Sharon McCskill, Retired Teacher, Lackland Elementary School, Lackland Air Force Base, San Antonio, Texas.

Doomed Path

I'm to reach a significant milestone which almost everyone strives to achieve – entering college. I've passed high school's threshold and am very soon entering college's campus, to join my fellow peers, hungry for knowledge, bright, embarking on a long road ahead of them. But this was not the road I had originally set upon at birth. My road was twisted, dark, and cut shorter than everyone else's.

I was born on May 31st, 2001 at Prince George Hospital, in Prince George County, Maryland. A few days after I was born, my parents reccived a letter which was a sad reminder that their attempt at constructing a new life would be set with tragic setbacks. Of course, they knew it would be hard – nothing was handed to them as they grew up. They clawed their way to their goals. This is a practically universal point of view for all immigrants – my parents were no exception. But expectation never really prepares you for the painful blow which reality deals. No matter how hard you brace yourself, you will still stumble back, a little winded, a little less stable. The letter stated that I had a disease called Sickle Cell Anemia.

My parents were born and raised in Kampala, Uganda, located in the Eastern part of Africa. While they didn't grow up with the luxuries I had at my disposal, they told me that they were still happy with their upbringing. Of course, it wasn't easy and they were eager to leave their home – as more opportunities lay outside their side of the fence. And they thought they would leave behind most, if not all of the misfortunes which befell Uganda. Of course, life was a cruel mistress, and she made sure they'd never forget their roots in one of the harshest ways possible: by striking their first born with Sickle Cell Anemia.

Sickle Cell Anemia is a blood disorder in which healthy red blood cells shed their flexible, circular-shape for that of a rigid, sickle-shape. The stiffness of the sickle-shaped cells leads to their blocking veins within the body, and preventing oxygen, as well as various, necessary nutrients from making their rounds about the body. Usually, this results in severe pain, often named a Sickle Cell Crisis. If not treated, conditions such as stroke can manifest, and one would most certainly die an early, and painful death.

My parents grew up in a society where Sickle Cell Anemia was as well-known as the common cold, though not met with the best reputation. If you were unlucky enough to have contracted Sickle Cell, you were met with little to no mercy. Most of the sick were abandoned by their parents, heckled, bullied, ostracized, and some did not have access to treatment. Those who did were better off, but still lived less than stellar lives. The most tragic aspect was that those who had Sickle Cell were guaranteed an early death, sooner or later in life. And they didn't have the proper help to at least ease their pain. They died slowly, in agony, looking to the sky with tired, jaundiced eyes, reaching for help with weak, pale hands, believing that they were cursed, as they had been told so their whole lives.

You had a 25% chance of contracting Sickle Cell if both parents have the trait, and all of this grief due to the 25% chance that your genetic makeup coded differently than a healthy individual still baffles me. It's the smallest things which can really topple over the biggest pyramids.

My being diagnosed with Sickle Cell horrified my parents – their plans to hit the ground running in chasing after their American Dream changed to an awkward waddling pace as they had to balance a sickly child atop both my parents working; my mother a nurse working in Intensive Care Unit and my father going to nursing school. It appeared we had been dealt a cruel hand, with my draw being the worst – I didn't even have a fighting chance, I was just a baby.

Texas

We hadn't moved to Texas until 2005, before then, my parents and I moved to Detroit, Michigan in 2001. That was where my younger brother Mark was born (thankfully healthy), and a choice encouraged by the Cord Blood Registry (CBR) themselves, his cord blood was harvested upon his birth, and stored for later use. Considering my health ailment, I figure my doctors thought that his cord blood could serve as some sort of use for me in the future, or perhaps it was the CBR themselves who came up with such a theory. But his cord blood will not resurface again until much later.

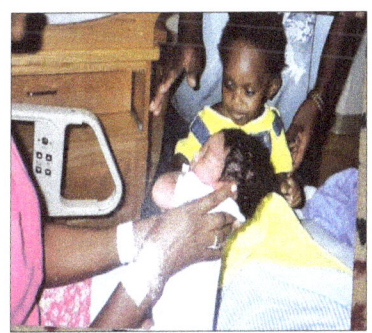

Excitement meeting my brother Mark

Mark is only two years younger than me, yet we act as if we weren't separated by even a day. Most of my childhood memories have him prominently beside me, whether that is with us intently watching Noggin, attempting to figure out how to pass a particular video game level, or simply building a fort with pillows, blankets, and table chairs we dragged to the living room.

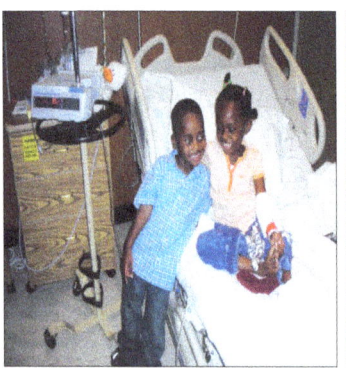
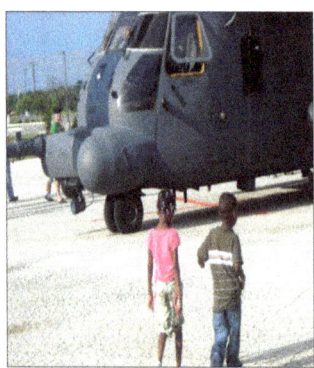

In a family home video recording the day of Mark's birth, when I first meet him, I am more so intent to grab hold of the chips on my mother's lunch tray than meet my new competition for parental attention. At some point, however, I grew fond of him and we became attached at the hip.

Sometime after Mark was born, my mother joined the United States Air Force, seeing it as one of the best options to give back to the country that gave her the opportunity to care for me, as this would have been impossible while in Uganda. Her first assignment was to Lackland Air Force

Base in San Antonio, Texas, and that's where it all began by the end of 2005.

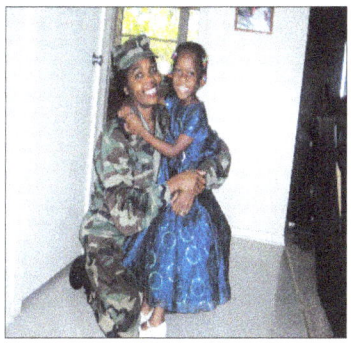

Much of what I can remember about my early childhood was while we were stationed at Lackland Air Force Base. I do not remember the move from Michigan to Texas, nor can I remember settling in and such into our one story, conjoined house. As far as I can recall, that house we lived in was essentially 'my first house.'

I did quite a bit of early growing in San Antonio – this is where I started Kindergarten, learned to ride a bike, had my first pet, got a new sibling, learned how to play the violin. Texas holds a special place in my heart, snuggled alongside all of the early memories I had cultivated while living there. I still miss it, even though I do love California just as much. And Texas is where the bulk of the story takes place.

Dr. Lockhart

I met my psychologist Dr. Lockhart at the end of 2006, and she was one of the most instrumental person in my life, as far as helping me cope with Sickle Cell. While I have little to no recollection of exactly how I came to know her, my mother said that it was through a doctor of mine, Dr. Major Howell, who we saw at Wilford Hall Medical Center at Lackland Air Force Base, who recommended her to us. According to her, the stress of having an inquisitive child with Sickle Cell was getting to her.

At five years-old, I was able to communicate with my parents whenever I experienced a Sickle Cell crisis, fatigue, or any other of the symptoms. However, I was also beginning to draw lines leading to conclusions which I could not understand, and so I turned to my parents, asking why I was the shortest in class; why the supposed-to-be whites of my eyes were more yellow than white compared to the other kids, Mark, my parents; why I was constantly in pain; why I was always in and out of hospital. I knew I wasn't living a normal life, it wasn't like the kids I saw on TV, or any of my classmates; heck, even my three-year-old brother who didn't even go to school yet had a much more normal life than I did.

Why, why, why, Mommy and Daddy? It's an innocent enough question, really. Anyone would want to know what was going on in their own body. But breaking the news of a life-threatening blood disorder to a child? That was too hard a task for my parents to bare in telling me. Explaining Sickle Cell meant explaining the various complications to come along with it – organ failure, stroke, death. Of course, they could hide it from me, I couldn't fully digest any of that I was only a kid; but you never feel good about hiding something this important from a child, do you?

So Dr. Lockhart came to my parents' assistance, gently coaching them on how to handle my questions concerning my health, not to mention soothe their own qualms of raising a sick child.

I don't remember my first visit with Dr. Lockhart, I don't remember many of them. But I remember her, a lady who I think was taller than or as tall as my mother at the time. She had warm brown eyes hiding behind a pair of glasses and a smile to match. I don't ever remember seeing her frown. I always felt safe and invited in her presence, and she didn't talk to me in a sort of condescending, fake tone which adults often used with kids. She appeared to be genuinely interested in what I had to say. My grandma was in that same way – I could hold full on conversations with her. I don't remember my mother being in the room whenever we had meetings – I think she was absent so that I wouldn't be afraid of holding anything back. The imposing figure of a mother can easily seal the lips of any child.

Dr. Lockhart broke the news to me of my condition, and I don't remember how I took it, but I believe it was a rather bewildered "Oh" not necessarily concerned with what it was. As long as I had a name to the cause then I was okay.

I remember during one of our first visits, she told me of how I could positively deal with my Sickle Cell through an imaginative exercise. I was to picture Sickle Cell as this monster, which I was then to loudly command to stay away from me, proclaiming that I wouldn't be its prey today. I was then to imagine putting it inside a cage, or even in the trash. I guess this exercise was meant for me to feel like I had control over the situation, that I could defeat this thing. That I had the controls, and it wasn't the other way again.

I remember later that night, while in my parents' room (I often slept with my parents despite having my own room), I sat up on my knees, stared at the door leading to their bathroom, and attempted to imagine a monster. I don't believe I had that good of an imagination as I usually took things at face value, so I simply said aloud "Go away, Sickle Cell!" My father questioned why I was doing that, to which I sheepishly responded that it was an exercise I was doing with Dr. Lockhart, and of course he understood and let me continue, but I suddenly felt very self-conscious about the whole thing and stopped. It felt silly.

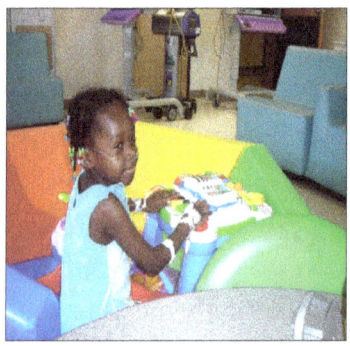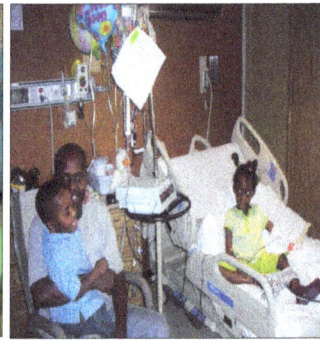

I never even imagined a 'monster' for the disease, though multiple times adults described it to me as the Sickle Cell Monster. Then and now I thought it a ridiculous, rather comical way to portray it, but any way to get the kids to grasp the concept would be fine. But I never thought it as a monster – I thought it for what it was: deformed, sickle-shaped blood cells blocking my veins, my chance at a normal life, and causing me pain. And not even Dr. Lockhart could sugar-coat it for me.

Ford's Funeral

I don't believe Dr. Lockhart introduced me to the concept of death, let alone the fact that there was a chance that I would die prematurely. I didn't have any major first-hand experiences with death around this time – the only experience I had were frogs getting run over near my house. Flat, dried pancakes which my brother and I would poke when my parents weren't watching. There was always a frog there, at that three-way intersection, and I thought it an interesting pattern.

But besides the death of the occasional amphibian, I had no personal experience with it. But I understood that when you died you wouldn't come back; that it was permanent. And that, for some reason, did not sadden or even frighten me. It was supposed to happen, I thought, so why be mad? It was inevitable, like the change from Cartoon Network to Adult Swim – I didn't like it, but it was supposed to happen, and I'd have to deal with it. Even when talking of my own death I was frank about it. Maybe I didn't fully understand its impact but I was rather frank when talking of the very real possibility my own, perhaps soon, passing.

In early 2007 I remember sitting in the living room with my mother, and the news was on, broadcasting the funeral of the late President Gerald R. Ford. I remember turning to my mother and asking, "Mommy, will that be me?" Taken aback, of course, she asked what I meant and I pointed to the casket – the centerpiece of the procession.

"In the casket."

Armed with the knowledge of my disease and its fatal implications, I basically asked "Am I going to die?"

It was a rather blunt question to me but something so much more heart-wrenchingly painful to my mother. I was only five, how could I understand that I was going to die sooner than most? And not only did I acknowledge it, but my mother was forced to, too. She was forced to look, if not for a brief moment, at the reality which I was presenting. The reality that her pride and joy, one of her first accomplishments in her life as an immigrant were not permanent.

I made her think about her having to bury me, not the other way around; of explaining to young Mark why I would no longer be home – if he'd even be able to remember me; of having to live day by day with the painful reminder that I had once cuddled in this blanket, ate from that plate, wore those shoes, and never would again. She didn't answer my question.

Hype

During one of my sessions with Dr. Lockhart, she sat me down by a low table in her office and drew out a purple stick figure with a crayon. She drew a large dot on its chest, and a lengthy line protruding away from its body. At the end of the line, she drew a square, and on the other side of the square, she drew two smaller lines branching off from one another. She drew a central line, and she explained, and this would be an instrumental tool in my Bone Marrow Transplant.

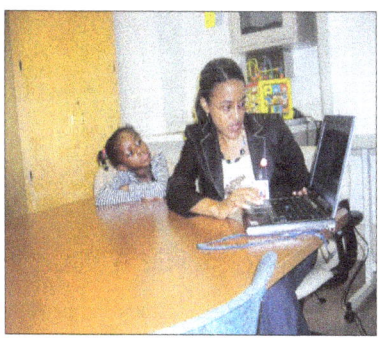

Dr. Lockhart during one of my sessions

I don't remember if she told me about the Transplant itself before or after the central line drawing, but at some point, she explained that I was getting a procedure which would eradicate Sickle Cell from my body, leaving me with a clean bill of health and free to do whatever I pleased. Of course, I was thrilled when she told me. I could be like all the other kids, not restrained by spontaneous pains, fevers, and such. I wouldn't have to miss so much school, I wouldn't have to be poked so often with needles, I wouldn't have to call the hospital home anymore, I wouldn't meet my casket so soon. I could finally be Sickle Cell free!

My parents had already made the decision some time beforehand and had asked Dr. Lockhart to relay the news to me. I readily accepted my chance at rebirth, however, as I kept asking when the transplant would be, I don't remember getting a definite answer. I was told sometime during the summer, then when school started, then a little after school started. I don't even remember being told what exactly was going to happen to me – what a Bone Marrow Transplant was, but the vague answers didn't bother me too much, I was just excited at the now very real prospect that I'd get to be cured, that freedom was so near within my reach.

In the meantime, I had another event to look forward to: the birth of my younger sister, Aliah. Mark and I picked out her name on a baby name website, and were thoroughly pleased that became her name. In hindsight, having a third baby while another child was beginning treatment probably wasn't the best choice if a clear-mind and lesser levels of stress were desired, but Aliah's arrival also added a nice light within our lives. We were running around, dazed, not entirely focused, that we forgot to cherish life, even with all of its warts. And despite her insistent, newborn wails, Aliah reminded us of that value.

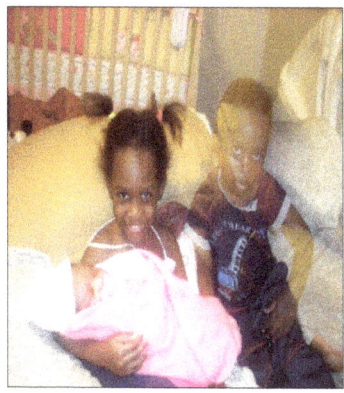

Two-Month School Year

I never formally finished second grade, as this was the year that my procedure took place in. I had only finished two years of schooling before I had to be pulled out. I was homeschooled for a short while in hospital and out – I'm hoping this large gap in my early school career does not affect my transcripts today.

There is a lovely picture of Mark and I on the first day of school – he was starting Kindergarten, and looked tiny with his larger backpack behind him. I hugged him tightly, making a huge show for my mother's camera, grinning widely. Mark did not look too thrilled for his first day or my affections.

My second grade teacher, Ms. Kay, was a very nice, very tall, bespectacled lady. I cannot remember most of the first day. I thought this classroom to be the oddest out of my previous two in that it appeared to be darker most of the time. We had windows, of course, I just remember the shades being drawn more often.

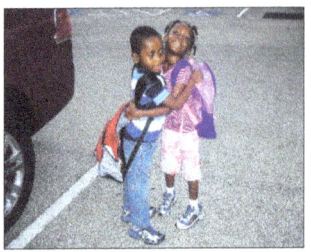

Mark and me

On that day, I either had to leave class early or perhaps stayed the whole day, but the point is that on my first day of Second grade, I went to Methodist Children's Hospital for an appointment. Methodist Children's Hospital is a Pediatric blood and Marrow Stem Cell Transplant center treating children, in San Antonio, Texas. It was near where I lived (about thirty minutes away I believe) and had the necessary equipment I would need for the transplant. I would come to know this place as home for the next few years. On this particular day, however, I met with one of my transplant doctors: Dr. Michael Grimley. He was a kind mind, his face always in a smile. Even his neutral look looked happy. And I was quite comfortable around him. I saw his face much more than I saw that of my second grade teacher's, as October rolled around, I had to leave second grade in order to go through with the Transplant, snuffing out what little memories I had of the classroom.

Two-Month School Year

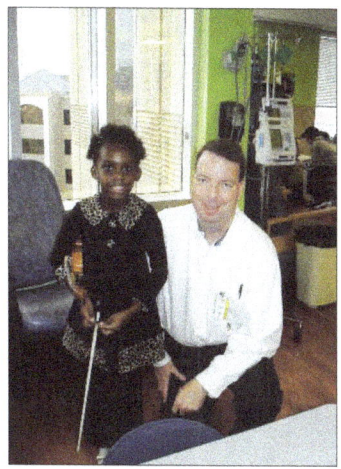

Dr. Grimley

Central Line Surgery

In preparation for the transplant, I had to get a Broviac central line implanted – for simplicity's sake, as well as the fact that I have always called the tube a central line, I will refer to it as a central line. A central line, as was explained to me, is a tube going into the heart, which protrudes out of your chest, splitting into two tubes which medicine can be received from. Mine had a blue, white and red tipped tube. This was the alternative to constantly being poked (as I loudly protested on many occasions).

Dr. Lockhart was the one to tell me that I would be getting a central line. During one of our visits she sat me beside the coffee table in her room, and took out a piece of paper. I don't remember exactly what she had said before drawing, but she explained to me that I would have to get a central line for my transplant. She drew a purple stick figure with a square on its chest to represent the dressing, or bandages covering the part protruding from the chest. A line branching off into two finished off the drawing. I had a simple explanation, visual and all and I wasn't nervous upon receiving one. I don't remember if I was told that I would receive it surgically though.

I had to leave early during school one day, and Ms. Kay gave me a sweet, sympathetic nod while I was walked off to the office for pick-up. I believe that it was my father who got me, driving me to Wilford Hall Medical Center which wasn't that far from school and known to me as a second home during my stay in Texas. I was checked in and settled into an in-patient room – I was used to that; I've had to stay overnight multiple times before.

The procedure was actually the next day, and I remember being woken up by my mother (she must've come earlier while I was asleep) and another nurse, who removed the nail polish from my fingernails. My mother gave me a bottle of dark magenta that I loved to paint on my bedroom wall, my dolls' faces, as well as my nails. She said I had pretty nails and was sorry that she had to remove them, but it was per guidelines for the surgery, and of course I was understanding about it all.

I was taken down to the surgery room, escorted by the nurse (or maybe a new one) and my mother. I was placed in a new bed outside the operating room – this was a sort

Central Line Surgery

of holding area for others waiting to go in I supposed. The nurse put on The Lion King for me while I waited, much to my delight. It was and still is one of my favorite classic Disney movies.

I remember a blur of nurses here, not one particular face, but someone had swung by to mark a particular place on my neck with a pen – and it tickled. The nurse explained that it was a marker for the surgeons, and assured me the mark would go away. A while later, another nurse gave me a dose of what they called 'laughing juice', or something like that. The name was to obviously soothe any fears I had about being put under, but I don't remember feeling fearful. The nurse told me that excessive laughter was a side effect, thus its name. Patients usually laughed before falling asleep. And I remember instantly bursting into fits of giggles after that. Looking back, I know I forced it, probably in the hope that such medication could make me laugh.

Before I was wheeled into surgery, my mother hugged me real tight, told me she loved me, and assured me I would be fine. I of course returned her affections, and assured her that I wasn't afraid. It was touching to have that moment before I was taken in – it's something I don't take for granted.

I remember being wheeled into the operating room before I was halfway through the movie, and I was beginning to feel weary, and my fake peals of laughter were growing weaker. The crowd of nurses surrounding me were warm and reassuring – I never felt the least bit uncomfortable. They told me that the laughing juice was making me sleepy, and I would be out like a light in a few seconds. While they bustled about me, I remember turning my head to the side, and seeing some painting on the wall ahead of me – I don't remember what it was, perhaps a bundle of balloons, or a cluster of clouds. Some comforting sight for jittery children going into surgery.

They put an oxygen mask over my nose and mouth, and I was out.

I awoke afterwards in a holding room for awaking patients, I assume. My mother was beside me, smiling widely. I think my father was there too, but I cannot recall, of course, as I was shaking off the effects of the anesthetic. I was groggy, disoriented – a given – and upset, for whatever reason. In the pictures taken of my recovery, I look completely miserable sitting next to my mother. I even refused to talk – I think I wished to just go back to sleep.

After recuperating for a little while I was wheeled back to my hospital room, and on the way back I remember passing by where I had been waiting to go into surgery – The Lion King was still on, and someone else was in my place, watching it. I felt a pang of jealousy.

Central Line Surgery

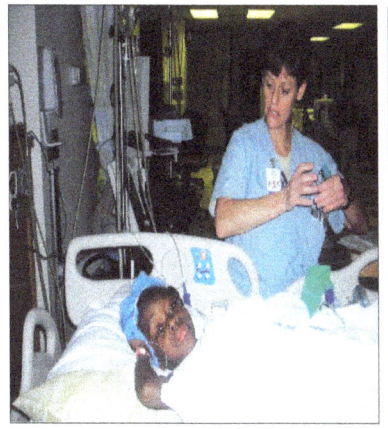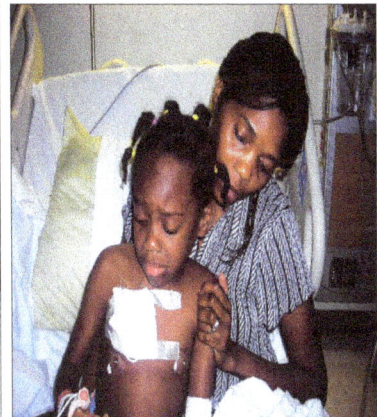

In the hospital room, they usually leave a coloring book in the barf basin for children. And there was a fresh copy when I returned, and I wanted it. But I still refused to talk, so I just pointed to it, hoping my mother would get the picture and fetch me the book. She did eventually.

After a while I slowly warmed up, finally talking when a doctor that I knew came in to check on me. Perhaps it was his cool-guy personality or the jokes he was cracking or something, but he got me to finally smile.

Following his visit, a small team of nurses came in next, wheeling in a portable X-ray machine. I had X-rays before, the ones where you stand in front of the board, lie on the table, even go through the huge machine itself – but I had never gotten one done by a portable one. I had to have the X-ray board lie across the bed, and I had to lie atop it. My shirt wasn't on – it hadn't been since coming out of the surgery; I don't think – and instead, I had a rather large patch of gauze. The board was so cold against my skin.

Eventually, Mark and Aliah came along with my father, and my aunt Bianca and her mother. I was delighted to see them all – my spirits were definitely lifted now. Mark came in with three fresh scratches above his cheek and, according to my father based on what Mark told him, he had been scratched by a fence at school. Later on, Mark told me he was scratched by a cat, and contended this story for the longest time before saying that he didn't know the true origin of the scars. Aunt Bianca had some strawberry shortcake bandages on hand which she gingerly placed over his scars. He didn't appear to be too bothered by it, honestly.

Around this time, I believe, a nurse who I had also come to know during my frequent visits came in and he cut me a little turtle neck vest-like thing out of a tube of netting most likely intended for medical use. That was to be worn over the central line, as support, so the tubes wouldn't be

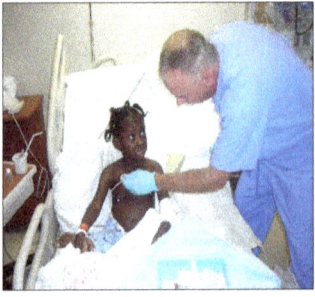
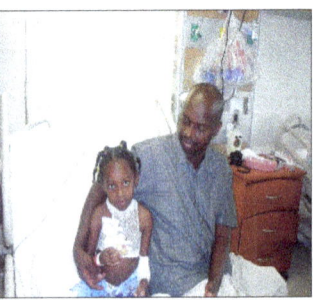

Central Line Surgery

hanging around while I went about my day. I'd come to know this familiar feeling, come to miss it when I no longer needed the netting.

I was warned to be very careful with the central line. I couldn't pull it, couldn't touch the site where it was protruding from my skin, couldn't get it wet, couldn't remove the dressing, etc. I was even given a small book about a little girl who also had a central line, mainly talking about how she was careful with it, made sure others didn't touch it, and wasn't hindered by it. I was very diligent about it, too, heeding their advice.

I have a funny story about the central line when I had gotten used to it. I was curious as to what it looked like, protruding out of my skin, so, in the privacy of my room, I had gently pried open a little bit of the dressing, just enough so that I could have a peek in but still be able to sufficiently close it. I remember seeing the line sticking out of my skin, and seeing small, black bundles of I don't know what surrounding the base. The sight was so weird and admittedly a little nauseating, and I quickly covered my tracks. I didn't repeat this until months later, this time not seeing the black stuff, but instead just seeing my skin seemingly growing onto the tube. It was so fascinatingly disturbing; it was skin-crawling. I never told my parents that I peeked.

Besides having to be careful when bathing (wearing a plastic bag around my chest) and wearing a netted turtle neck, I also had to get used to the daily maintenance of my central line. Since this tube was delivering medication and had direct access to vital veins in my body, it was paramount that it was cleaned daily, to avoid serious infection.

Performed during my hospital stay at Methodist Children's Hospital and while at home, a nurse or my parents (usually my mother who is also a nurse) would have to carefully do my dress changes following the orders of my doctor, and with a specifically medicated sponge, would clean around the area of which it was attached. The first couple of times, I just about squirmed at this part. It just felt so weird – so cold and wet, like some sick dog's tongue. Then, the tubes had to be flushed out. One tube had a white end cap and would be flushed out with a clear solution in a black labeled syringe, and the other had a red end cap, flushed with a yellow labeled syringe. This was the most curious feeling to me – I could feel the cool rush of liquid entering me. I never liked that and it was my least favorite part. Afterwards, a clean dressing was applied.

All of this maintenance was done while I was lying down, staring up at the ceiling or at whoever was doing the cleaning. They had to wear gloves, face mask and had to be careful not to breathe or spit on me. It wasn't long before the cleaning became routine, and I memorized every part of it.

Central Line Surgery

I was never really worried about the central line appearing as a bump underneath my clothes until my mother pointed it out herself, wondering if any of the other kids would point it out. I went to school self-conscious about whether or not the bump was visible, if anyone pointed it out. And a few kids did point it out, but I explained what it was. The whole class knew that I had some sort of medical condition – I assume Ms. Kay told them at the behest of my parents – and everyone was quite understanding, and I was never treated differently. I went to school and played about as if I hadn't gotten a tube implanted in my chest. I forgot that it was there most of the time, too. My second skin, as I now affectionately call it.

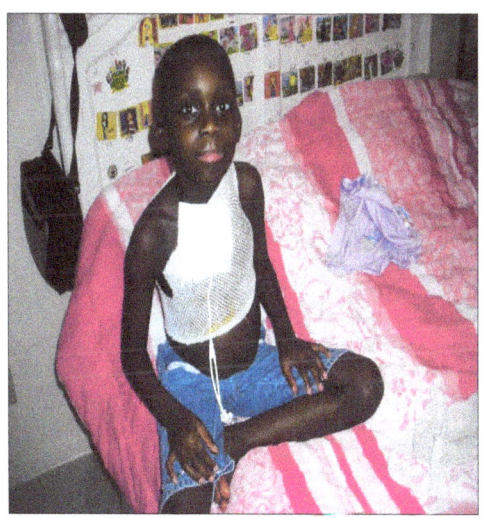

Just Like Home

I am terrible with dimensions, and I cannot remember the exact size of my hospital room. All I can really say of it is that it was perhaps the largest one I have ever occupied (of course, it was still rather small). Right outside the door there was a sink and it was required that you wash your hands before you entered – no exceptions. In preparation for my Bone Marrow Transplant, my immune system would be left extremely weak, and I would be easily susceptible to infection. However, I forgot about the constant threat of sickness during my stay. I was distracted by the window.

A few feet away from the left side of my hospital bed stood the only window in the room – it provided all of the natural light and gave me a view of what I was missing, which was construction on the hospital and nearby traffic. It was quite a large window, too – perhaps two and a half feet of wall raising from the top and bottom while the pane took up the rest of the space. There was a little seat where you could perch in front of the window, too. I spent quite a bit of time looking out that window, excited at first that I got such a nice view – but I quickly grew bored of it. It was like a window seat of a plane – it's nice at first but it's just an extensive, unchanging sea of clouds for the most part.

In front of my hospital bed, mounted on the wall, I had a TV. The best part about this, I remember, is that it could play DVDs as well as change to satellite – usually, I had a box television set rolled into my room with VHS tapes and while I did like the selection, it didn't have the variety which satellite did. I also remember that my mother allowed me to watch Disney Channel, as it was the only kids' program airing at night, and I often stayed up. Methodist Children's Hospital was where I consumed much of my childhood Disney Channel content without the worry of my parents telling me to switch it off.

My IV pole and vitals were on the right side, as where mostly everyone who came into the room stood – on the right side. I don't remember many people standing on the left side of the bed. My bed itself was dressed in my own bedsheets from home, just for added hominess.

Farther away on my right side, at the wall of the room, there was a second bed where my parents slept during their shifts to watch me. Between us was a small nightstand, mini-fridge, radio, and portrait of my family which my mother brought – so I wouldn't forget anyone's faces, and not miss them too much. There was an attached bathroom, too, and I remember an incident in which I had to go but didn't want to wake my mother up, as it was night time. So I tried moving the heavy IV pole myself and heading to the bathroom – there was a reason I needed assistance, it was so heavy! And I had an accident right there and after a couple of nurses came in and cleaned up my mother tiredly told me that it was alright if I woke her up. I was potty-trained, thank goodness, and also polite.

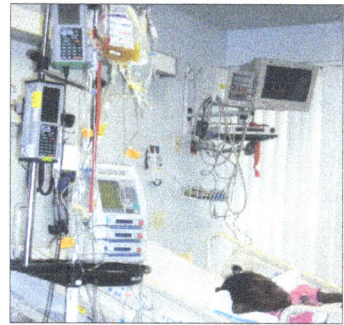
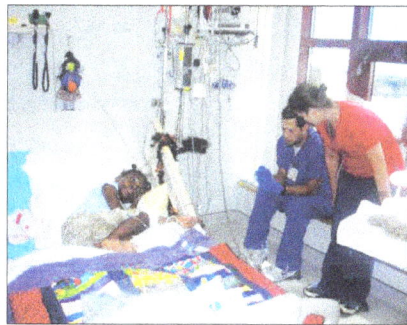

When I first moved into the hospital room, my aunt Bianca and her mother came in bearing decorations to liven up my room. I was delighted that they were there and even more so that they came with gifts. As it was autumn, they got me a small witch holding a pumpkin which was hung above my bed, and a large, paper figure of a scarecrow was hung on my closet. A feeding tube was later hung in front of that as part of a later campaign to get me to eat.

Later on during my stay, I got a toy kitchen moved in and I was reminded of the one I had in my own room back home. It had a dozen plastic foods, pots, and pans that I rarely used. I think it was my mother who requested for it. And a good move, too. That's what I went for to even get out of bed most of the time. Reaching for a bit of home. And it was easy for me to ease into calling this room home – I'd been doing so for the past seven years, and this was no different.

Hospital Anecdotes

Being stuck in a hospital for a medical procedure didn't mean that I could slack off on moving about. And I had no excuse since I was a kid. I had regular visits from multiple physical therapists while in Methodist Children's Hospital, and they were some of the kindest, most encouraging people I have ever met.

One of the nurses was a very kind lady who would sometimes mention the comical antics of her grandchildren. She helped me decorate my hospital room within my first couple of weeks, and made me feel quite at home. As home as I could feel, at least. I sorrowfully regret that I had forgotten her name. In fact, the name of most of my caretakers have left me, and I haven't seen most of them since my visit back in 2012. However, very recently, I was reunited with one of my nurses, nurse Kendra who was being oriented by my main transplant nurse Dallas, at a baby shower.

One day, nurse Dallas had brought me a paper with stars and angels which I colored in, cut out, and pasted on the windows. She helped me hang up a banner which my classmates had sent me – one which said *Feel Better, Carol!* And I sadly do not know where that banner is. She placed my get well cards on the window sill of the window, suggested where I placed multiple decorations I received – I rarely saw my room as a hospital room, as cliché as it sounds. I viewed it as any other room, really. And that made my extended stay all the more comfortable.

* * *

In preparation for the transplant, as previously written, I had to take several doses of Chemotherapy, a severely strong, not to mention weakening drugs. The waning effects of Chemo plus my having to stay indoors were definitely diminishing my previous strength. And I needed to preserve that strength, not to mention build up more in my reserves, in order to go through with the transplant without any issues. And that is where my physical therapists come in.

They had multiple activities for me to do involving my standing, stretching, pushing, whatever that may be. It wasn't strenuous activity, and I would certainly take this over running a track any day.

One activity I remember was where I had to sit down and use one foot to push a slipper which the therapist had grasped between their hands, or wedged between their legs. It may seem like an easy task, and it sounded like it to me – but it wasn't. Maybe I was going soft or maybe the therapist was using more strength than I could fight, but it took me quite a while before I could release my slipper from their grasp. And my leg ached a little afterwards.

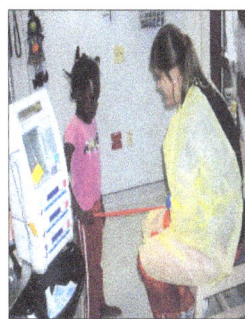
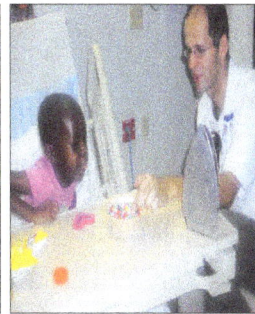
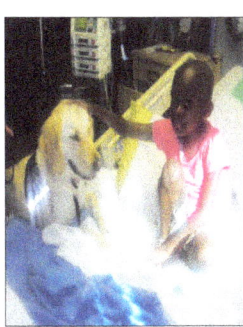

I did other activities such as bowling with foam balls and plastic pins, stretching with rubber strips and such. I was always encouraged to move about my room every day, to bend fully when picking items up – making sure I wasn't utilizing the time to be cooped up inside to be totally inactive.

* * *

Despite my being isolated in the hospital, I did receive visitors from the outside. One frequent visitor was my first grade teacher, Ms. McCaskill, who kept in touch with my mother and would sit by my bedside.

We often watched 'The Lion King' whenever she arrived – it became a ritual at some point. Every time Ms. McCaskill would come to visit, one of my parents would pop 'The Lion King' in the VHS player and I'd relive the story of Simba and his coming of age to be king over and over. I never got tired of it. At some point, Ms. McCaskill brought the soundtrack she had for the film, lending it to me to listen to at my leisure – my mother remembered to bring in my radio from home and while I never really listened to it, she would always play a CD from home and lightly dance with me in the room.

I don't remember watching 'The Lion King' without Ms. McCaskill bring present, and with the coming of the remake, I like to remember how often I had watched the original.

* * *

One effect of Chemotherapy which I was most excited for was losing my hair – I was told that I would eventually end up bald and I took the news quite well. I'd be like Calliou, a brat who I actually didn't mind at the time. And it would be a fun look to try on!

I started losing my hair slowly, bits of it coming out when it was brushed, mini bald patches manifesting on my skull. At some point, and I don't remember how this came to be, I yanked out a large tuft of hair, with the hair tie still attached. It left half of my skull in an awkward, patchy pattern, and the other half relatively covered.

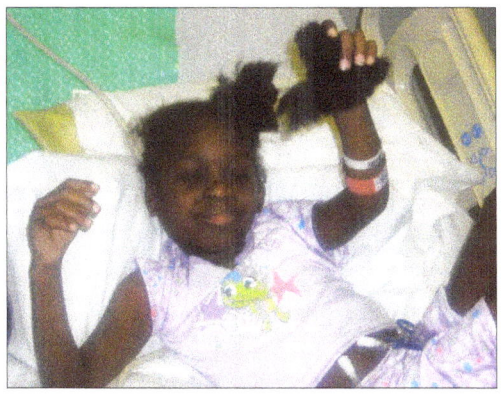

At some point, I'm assuming my doctors didn't want me to keep yanking my hair out, a barber came in to shave the rest of my hair. For some reason, I thought this would hurt, or be terribly uncomfortable, so I cried as she began shaving my head. My mother held me during the ordeal, attempting to smile for the camera as I made it out to be much worse than it was. Of course, when she was finished, I was totally amused by my baldness that I forgot about how terrified I was of the razor.

I was given several hats meant to wrap around my head and tie at the back in various designs which I have long lost, but it was a new addition to my closet that I only wore outside, as I was I wanted to flaunt my lack of hair for as long as I could. Before it grew back within a few months, of course.

Blue Smiles

Over the course of my stay in Methodist Children's Hospital, my behavior changed, and not for the better. Most of the time, I was bright, bubbly, talkative, antsy to do anything – as any normal child would be. Sickle Cell didn't damage that aspect of me. And even the somber setting of a hospital – let alone a children's one – didn't dampen my mood.

I remember making great friends with the nurses, always having a story to tell them, asking what all they were administering to me that day – I even talked about Disney's Sleeping Beauty, and we had a friendly debate over her name being Aurora and not actually Sleeping Beauty as I always thought; and how I had never seen it with one of the nurses. Surprised, she lent me her copy of Sleeping Beauty and I watched it. I didn't think much of the movie; I knew the story already.

However, as I had my ups, I had my downs. And something wore me down, and I'm not sure what. My consistent, chipper self slowly degraded. The smile was becoming too heavy to wear. My parents noted on my Caring Bridge website that I had days where I appeared to be depressed, remaining quiet and gloomy, and my mother commented on my apparent change in behavior upon her recollection.

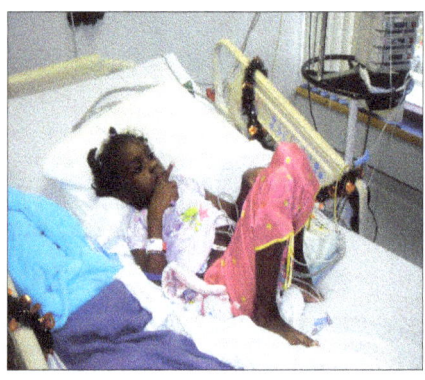

There were times when I didn't feel like engaging with my physical therapists, nurses, even my parents. I didn't want to play on the laptop, I didn't even want to watch TV. I didn't want to do anything; I was just tired. I wanted to be alone, to perhaps curl myself up in a makeshift cocoon out of the blankets, and shut myself out from everyone else, even if it was just for a little while. Of course, I was not given the luxury of privacy as someone was always present to watch me.

I remember how at some point during my stay, I no longer wanted to eat. My appetite decreased. Of course, I still ate, just not a healthy amount for a sick child; I just wasn't that hungry anymore. I refused to eat whatever meal was served to me, whether it be from the hospital cafeteria, or even McDonalds, a favorite of mine. One time, a therapist of mine came to visit me, and tried to coax me into eating some rice my mother brought from home. I ended up breaking down for no reason and she took my hands in hers and looked me in the eye and gently told me of how important it was that I ate and eating would help with my recovery and etc. I ate a few bites – they went down harshly in my throat.

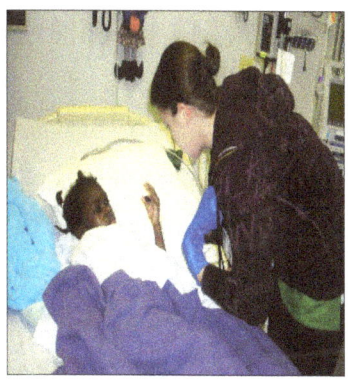

At the time, food smelled really weird to me, just unappetizing. And it even hurt to eat at times – at one point, I grew white rings on the side of my tongue and sores all over my mouth which had to be rinsed out with a lidocaine type saline solution. I am unsure of how or why they developed, or if they were related to my refusal to eat or due to chemotherapy.

I remember my mother kept telling me that if I continued this route of pushing away food, I'd have a feeding tube implemented. She described it in such a grotesque manner that I felt tingly whenever I pictured myself with a feeding tube. I only adhered to my mother's warnings and forced myself to eat once she had a nurse hang a feeding tube, still packaged, in my hospital room, right under the TV, in clear sight for me to see. Scare tactics work.

In addition to my refusal to eat, there were days where I was upset for no reason. I refused to smile, and would rather not talk to anyone. So I would simply remain in my bed, staring up at the TV, the wall, the window, not really in the mood for any communication. It really bugged me when people would try to coax me to talk, asking for a smile or even a little story. I was just so tired of it all – couldn't I have one day where I could be left alone?

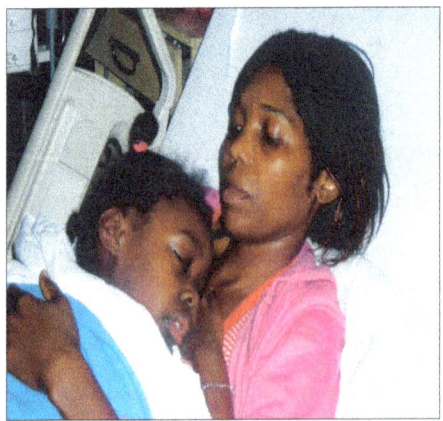

I don't know what wore my enthusiasm down. Maybe it's the fact that I was a child, forced into staying in a room for a large amount of time, tethered and unable to leave. I never felt like a prisoner, but I certainly didn't want to stay there. I knew this was for my own good, that I would feel better after all of this. But I was worn out from the illness, the medication, the needles, being cooped up. I could see the street from my large window, but even the majority of the hospital took up most of the view. Is captivity made even more unbearable with the presence of windows? I believe so.

Drumroll Please:
The Bone Marrow Transplant

I was generally kept out of the loop in regards to how long my stay would be, when changes in my care would be implemented, and so on. Actually, in regards to such routines, I cannot recall much of anything. Various snippets deemed memorable during my stay are all I can remember. Of course, I did spend most of my days bored out of my mind, trying to occupy myself with TV, the internet, or whatever else, all while waiting for the anticipated procedure which was to save my life.

I do not remember if a calendar was kept in my room, and if there was one, I don't think I checked it often. In fact, I cannot recall if I was told about the transplant's date, how long it would be, and so on. I do not even remember bopping about the room in earnest, waiting for the transplant day to arrive. As with just about everything else that I had to endure, I felt rather indifferent to the procedure.

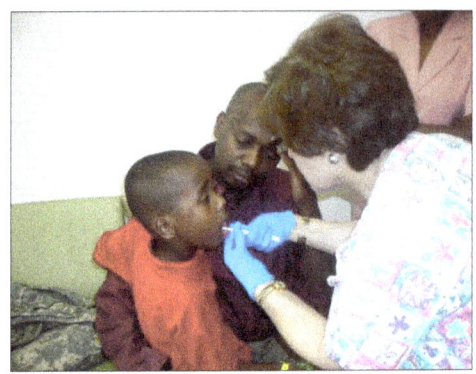

Mark's DNA and HLA tying

But I digress; October 30th, 2008 came with the arrival of most of my family. For about two and a half months, I haven't seen Mark or Aliah and was obviously excited to reunite. However, I quickly took notice of my insufferable five-year-old brother's absence. My parents had gone down to the operation room earlier as comfort for him as he was about to go into surgery to donate his bone marrow.

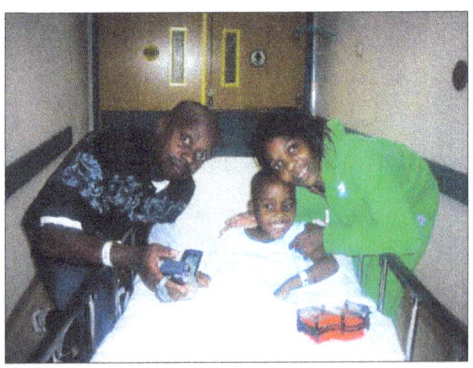

Drumroll Please: The Bone Marrow Transplant

I don't recall receiving an explanation for the empty seat, but if I did, it must've been an explanation that today was my transplant day. The excitement that today was the day in which all of the medication and time spent in the hospital away from family away from a normal childhood had led up to fell short with me.

Oddly enough, I do not feel much of a swell of dizzying joy at that I was getting cured. Perhaps I was too young to really appreciate the gift which they were siphoning out of my brother, or maybe it is my current, perpetually angry adolescent mind which is snuffing out all of the warmth from the memory. That is to say, I am still grateful that the transplant happened in the first place, or this book will have taken a drastically different turn. Perhaps it'd be a chapter or two shorter, the end cut short just like the author.

Anyway, I cannot remember sharing the same excitement as the rest of the adults around me did. I was more so one step closer to my bewildered sister, wondering why she wasn't getting as much attention as she usually did. And I cannot recall how exactly I spent the rest of my morning but later on, perhaps some time in the afternoon, my dazed brother Mark was wheeled into my hospital room. I was delighted to see him, but he was far too inebriated by anesthetic to truly comprehend what was happening. In fact, if you look at all of the pictures he is in on this day, he looks sleepy or upset.

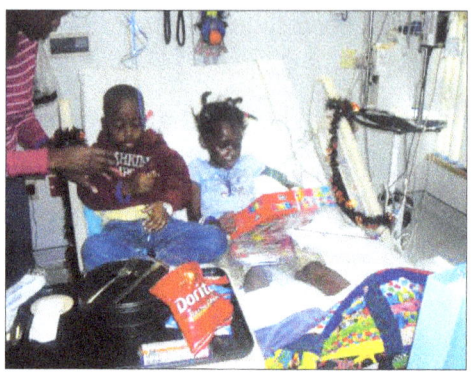

I remember him being helped into my hospital bed, and oddly enough, I felt a strange, uncomfortable tingle ripple through me as he was in such close proximity. For whatever reason, I felt irked by his loopy state. Of course, I was still happy to see him. But Mark wasn't much for conversation and I unfortunately could not pass the time in discussing current cartoons we had seen, his progress on multiple PS2 games, or even how home and school were. And as much as I wanted to catch up, I left him alone to his out-of-it state.

Everyone else in the room – family and nurses alike – buzzed with joy, filling the room with excited chatter. The energetic commotion was enough to make me dizzy, and it probably blotted out most of my memory of this day. Unfortunately, I cannot even remember when the blood containing my brother's extracted bone marrow was wheeled into my room – my key to getting rid of these genetic shackles.

Funny story, I remember glancing out of the small window affixed to the door of my hospital room, allowing

Drumroll Please: The Bone Marrow Transplant

me to see a rectangular strip of hallway. I saw a bundle of blue and yellow balloons and a small part of me wished that I was the recipient of the balloons. I got blood, not balloons, seven-year-old me thought dejectedly.

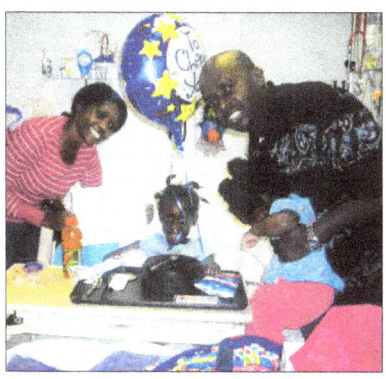

A certificate congratulating me

However, in the midst of the excited commotion, the door opened and two nurses came in carrying those balloons, along with a bundle or gifts. Now I matched the adults' joy, although for varying reasons.

At some point, on 29th October 2008 the bag containing Mark's bone marrow was hooked up to my central line, and for the first time in my life, I was receiving blood instead of having it extracted. On 30th October the next day a small bag of cord blood was also infused into my central line. I think there was a thick hush which set about the room, killing all talk from before. My father had the camera ready, the TV was either muted or off, all eyes were on my brother and I.

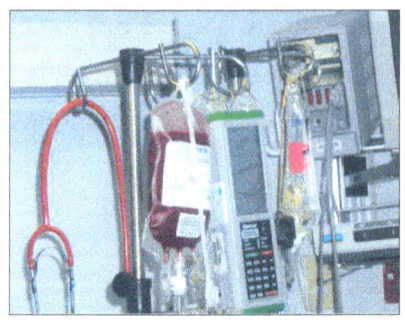 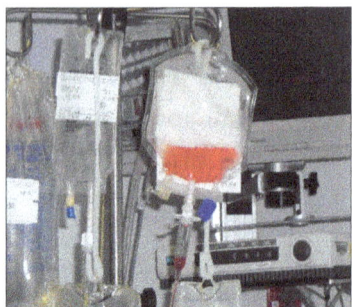

Mark's bone marrow bag   *Mark's cord blood bag*

As a child, whenever you hear adults making such a fuss over something, you expect it to be quite the spectacle. I learned then and later on that a Bone Marrow Transplant was a procedure in which marrow would be extracted from a donor's hip or thigh bone (in this case, my then 4 year-old little brother Mark's femur) and then transplanted into the recipient. The point of receiving doses of Chemotherapy was to kill off the sickled cells which were already causing me trouble, and to suppress the immune system, so that the new blood cells would not be attacked, thus leading to a violent rejection.

However, when the bone marrow transplant was being described to me, the excited tone which every adult used made me think it some spectacular thing to happen, some astonishing show, of the likes I couldn't comprehend. But seeing that the highlight of the day was simply receiving blood through a tube (which I have been doing for my whole life with medication) made me perceive the

Drumroll Please: The Bone Marrow Transplant

transplant as underwhelming. Really, another prolonged hospital visit.

Whilst the blood slowly flowed into my system, I went to work in tearing into what I was really interested in – the presents. While I may have received more, all I remember getting was some sort of sand play set, in which you had multiple packets of colored sand which could fill differently shaped plastic bottles. To make interesting lines in the sand, an included stick could be used to stab into the sand filled bottles and make cool designs. I remember playing with that set a few days later, but I never saw that sand set again. Mark got a huge nerf gun, which he would have been bouncing off the walls if he hadn't gotten out of surgery beforehand.

The rest of that day was spent with me awkwardly posing with my family, with my balloons, my toys – the blood bag got its own photoshoot. I got multiple congratulations but couldn't understand what there was to congratulate about. Soon after, as the day came to a close, I had to bid goodbye for now to Mark and Aliah. I was particularly crushed to see them go, as we hadn't even been together for a whole day, but was assured that I could visit them soon. And maybe that's when the ability of the bone marrow transplant hit me.

The whole reason why I had left school, underwent central line placement surgery, taken doses of chemotherapy, been holed up in my hospital room shut away from anything and everyone else I knew was so I could walk out a different kid. I had walked in, sickly and in need of help, and I would walk out healthy, strong and proud to cheat death. I could go back home, go back to school, maybe even get a pet as my parents promised; could do all I ever wanted to do without this ticking, biological ball and chain clinging onto me. This was my savior, I knew, even as a seven-year-old girl who was far too interested in toys earlier. I was ecstatic to leave and embrace the world with fresh arms, fresh eyes – a fresh life. I like to say that October 30th, 2008 is my second birthday for that very reason.

Indoor Trick-or-Treating

No one bothered to explain the recovery process to me. All of the adults were too excited to really pay attention to anything else – poor Mark suffered later that night when he complained about ants biting the extraction point on both his hip, and my parents realized that they forgot to give him pain killers.

The transplant was described to me as this miracle cure, with overnight results. To the young mind of a child, I interpreted the explanations as the transplant being an instant cure-all, a magic elixir. I'd soak up my brother's blood and the disease which I'd been riddled with would instantly fade from my system. I would be rid of all my pain, I could grow, I could go to school, I could get out of the hospital! No more Sickle Cell, no more problems! I'd be outta there before they could unhook my central line from the IV pole.

However, the young mind of a child usually does not understand the agonizingly slow pace in which recovery takes. My hopes had been raised for an exciting, instant cure, and I had been let down twice.

I remember expecting to leave the hospital room the day after the transplant, maybe I could even go back to school next week at the latest. All I got were late congratulations and a bag of Mark's frozen stem cell blood, harvested from his umbilical cord when he was newly born, at the suggestion of Dr. Shurney (Pediatric Hematologist-Oncologist, Children's Hospital, Michigan), figuring that it could perhaps help me sometime in the future. The purpose of his banked stem cells was to replace cells which had been destroyed by chemotherapy, such as white blood cells, as cord blood cells can take the form of any cell dependent on where in the body it is introduced.

The next day was Halloween, and I spent it walking five doors down to the playroom where various other children in my shoes as well as their parents hovered over their shoulders, peering behind their IV poles. I wore a Sleeping Beauty dress, having recently watched the Disney movie for the first time as a nurse lent her copy of the movie to me, surprised that I hadn't seen it yet. I was accessorized with a matching tiara, wand, and medical mask. Instead of trick-or-treating as Mark and Aliah got to do, I colored small pumpkins along with the other children. I was still too sick to eat candy.

I appeared to be politely miserable in the photos which my father had snapped that day, but I do not remember feeling much remorse at not being able to go trick-or-treating. Sure, I would rather have been in festively decorated neighborhoods rather than the crowded room of a hospital playroom, but I didn't complain much. Later on, I was brought fried chicken in my hospital room, and wore a face-splitting smile for the camera my father held. I don't think I ate the chicken.

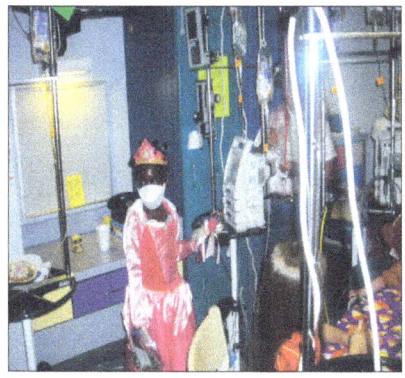

This Halloween celebration I had to spend indoors rather than out despite having received my supposed miracle beforehand was perhaps my first clue into the fact that I wasn't done yet, and I still had a long way to go. I only wish someone had explicitly told me about the recovery process, before I had let my hopes run too far. By how everyone was describing it, I really thought I would go home the very next day.

I found out later that I would have to remain in the hospital even after my transplant, and this part of the stay was where I began to get restless. I fell into this brief spiral of exaggerated childhood melancholy, wondering if I was to ever be cured, and thinking that this whole procedure was all for naught. I would still have Sickle Cell; everything the nurses would do would fail; I would die before I got to go home, which was just something I really wanted to do. At least let me play one more game with my brother again.

I was agitated that I was to remain here under the pretense of untold false hope, yet excited that once I did return, I got to act like a normal kid. Surely the effects of Sickle Cell would have been fully eradicated, and the transplant would have worked its magic, right? Of course not. Recovery was a long road that I did not have the patience to drive.

Temporary Solace

Sometime after my transplant, I was told the wondrous news that I could go home on a pass!

For a visit. I hadn't been home in about two and a half months, maybe more maybe less, I hadn't kept track of the time. I had a large picture of my family – my parents, Mark, Aliah, and I, garnished with a blue, curly bow in my hospital room, and that was a constant reminder of what I was missing out on. I had briefly talked on the phone with my siblings a few times, but it wasn't the same as being in the same room as them; I hadn't seen my siblings since the transplant by this point and I was aching to see them once more, not to mention getting out of the hospital at long last.

I was to wear a hat to protect (or perhaps hide?) my bald head, as well as a mask to ward off infection. These were my essential accessories during this part of my recovery, where

I was allowed to venture outside. They never clashed with my outfit and I was quite the fashionista back then, more so than I am now.

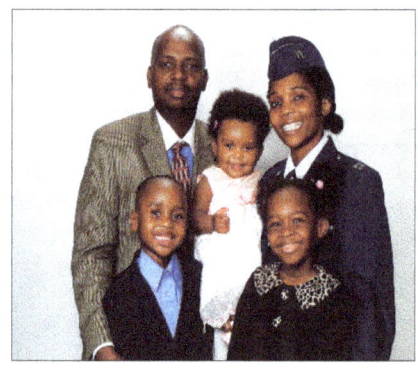

The day of my first visit, one of my parents (I don't remember who took me home) stopped by Burger King before driving me home. Nothing had changed much about the house since I had left, but I was pleased, regardless. Aliah regarded me as if I were a stranger – and I didn't blame her. I had been absent for quite some time, and I doubted that she was old enough to make connections as to who I was. She was more interested in the food.

Mark was excited to see me (at least, that's how I remember it) and that warmed my heart. He was the one kid close to my age who I had spent the most time with my whole life – we shared favorite cartoons, cereals – we even learnt how to ride bikes at the same time. I was aching for another child to talk to and he was right here. Mark was playing our PlayStation 2 when I came to visit – it was either some Sonic the Hedgehog game, or Ratchet and Clank, both of which I don't think we ever finished. And, tragically enough, our PS2 had met its end when Aliah decided to pour orange juice all over it, thus rendering our favorite games – such as Over the Hedge, based off of the movie, and this Disney princess one I had fancied myself – utterly useless. We still haven't quite forgiven her for it.

Mark allowed me a few turns on the game, whatever it was, but he mostly took control. In fact, I don't remember us talking much during my visits. Of course, my parents would prod us into conversation, saying: "Aren't you happy your sister is home?" or something along the lines of that. Fodder for the video camera.

Mark, years later, told me that due to my extended absence, he had forgotten that he even had an older sister. I'm not sure if he said so to be dramatic or if he was genuine. Considering how young he was, I do not think he was exaggerating. I don't know what he was told in regards to my absence, what explanation he was given. But to think that I had been sponged from his memory due to only a few months' absence leaves a bitter taste in my mouth. To think that my longing for my brother was one-sided, that he didn't even bat an eye at my absence while I was nearly bawling my eyes out at being away for so long. And of course Aliah didn't have the slightest clue of what was going on – she was only a year old.

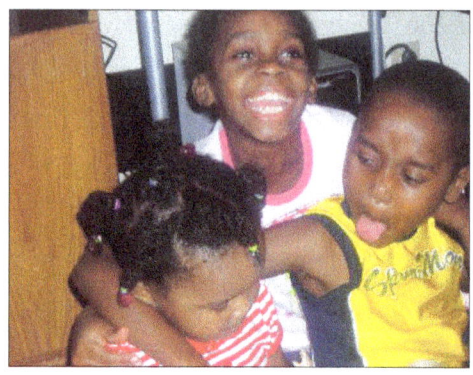

But I was enjoying my time away from the hospital and at home, here with my family, all together as it should be. I had yearned for this for so long, and I finally got what I wanted. I was satisfied. I didn't care that I was bald, or that I couldn't go outside without a mask and hat, and I didn't mind all of the time spent in the hospital cut away from my childhood as I had before. I was home, and that was all that mattered.

I was devastated when my mother told me that I'd have to go back to Methodist. I wouldn't be sleeping in my own bed tonight. I bid Mark and Aliah good-bye, and went back to my second home.

I was granted another visitation pass, I assume to see if I was still stable from my first, and it played out much like before, with me sitting beside Mark, playing video games. In fact, the visits are so similar that they have melded into one in my memory. I can't recall any details distinguishing one visit from the other. All I can say is that I got to venture outside of what I knew as home for the last couple of months, and return to my real one.

More time had passed (my guess is about a few weeks after) and I was told that I could go home – not as a visit, but permanently. My doctors concluded that my immune system was stable enough to leave the sterile conditions of Methodist and return to the less sterile conditions of my home.

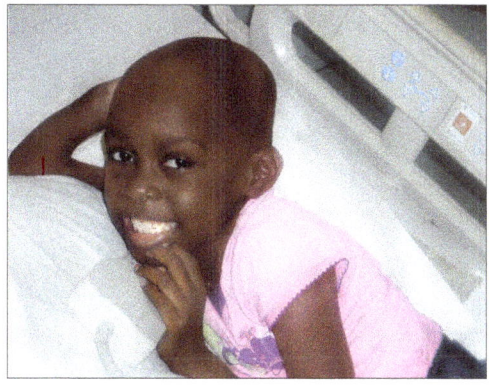

My parents drove me home, and I remember holding an ironed craft I had done with one of the child life specialists. It was one of the first activities we ever did together – a heart made of beads ironed together – and I had that clutched in my fist as we made our way to their car. I can't remember the exact way my last day in Methodist panned out – I don't even remember what the hallways, nurses station, or even the outside of the hospital itself looked like. But I didn't care at that point – I didn't look back. All I cared about was that I could finally be outside my window– I could be the construction workers, the cars, the birds.

All that silent weeping I did at not being able to go home; that painful yearning to just put my head down on my own pillow, just to glimpse my house for even a second – it wasn't in vain. I could finally say goodbye to the room I had known has home for the past few months. The transplant was finally working the magic which all the adults gushed about and I could finally go home.

Home but Not Yet Free

Even when I returned home, it was as if I hadn't left the hospital, in that I was forced into a rigorous routine of constant cleanliness: I had to wash my hands frequently, along with the rest of my family; my bed sheets had to be changed often – sometimes twice a day; my room and personal bathroom were regularly sanitized; my clothing was washed constantly; our carpeting in the house had to be removed prior to my leaving the hospital. I couldn't hug my siblings without being fearful of contracting illness – my immune system was still weak. I couldn't go outside, I couldn't have flowers, pets, or even strawberries: all of which was to prevent serious infection in compromising the recovery process. Catching a simple cold, I was told, could land me into the hospital in intensive care. Looking back, I wonder if this was another embellished warning so that I wouldn't be reckless.

Of course, there was no room for me to be reckless with my recuperating health. Both my parents were nurses and understood the importance of cleanliness in relation to health, especially in patients with weak immune systems such as myself. And young children were especially at risk. They took on the role of the team of nurses who watched over me while at the hospital. They made sure that every surface I was to sit upon was spotless. They even explained to me how important it was that I kept clean and healthy, and of course I would listen to such scary, imposing figures as my parents. I didn't want to spend another extended stay at the hospital, let alone upset my parents.

And it was easy for me to abide by a strict, clean regiment – I was used to it. I don't remember how I spent most of my time at home, but if I had to take a guess, I probably stayed in my room all day watching television. My sanitized toys were paramount to me at this time. Actually, were my toys sanitized? Or had they been given to Aliah, or tossed? I don't remember the fate of most of my toys.

And even though I was back home, I felt there was no change. My room was indeed my own – I knew this bed, broken from when I jumped about on it; this dresser, decorated with every sticker I had received after each blood drawing; this pink princess castle bookcase, something I had gotten through miscommunication on my own part. I told my mother I wanted a pink princess castle, one which I saw in a newspaper ad: it was a tent. The bookcase was a gift, and came with four Disney princess stickers, and I liked it all the same. I was afraid of this room at first, I still slept with my parents when we moved in, I think. I refused to leave them. They were my safety, and to leave my parents' room would mean certain death.

One day, I received a package from my second grade classmates. To be honest, I had forgotten about most of them – except Jacob, of course – and I was sure I had slipped from their mind. I left at the beginning of the school year after all, surely they couldn't reach that far back to remember my face?

I think my mother must've been keeping tabs with Ms. Kay, and she decided it would have been a great morale boost to receive a present from my class, and what a boost it was. And unfortunately, as delightful as the gift was, I cannot remember most of its contents. I cannot even remember if I got a card, although I'm sure I had. All I can remember was a red, plastic Crayola case with colored paper, coloring pencils, crayons and other art supplies. I hadn't used that case for a few months until one night, I randomly awoke, took out a paper and pencil, doodled, and pasted it on my wall. All of the paper was used up almost immediately after that. A bit of color to my usually off-white walls. My room did remind me of the hospital anyway.

Baby Steps

While Halloween was the first holiday I spent after my transplant, Thanksgiving was the first holiday I spent with my family, relatively Sickle-Cell free. The night before, my siblings and I prepared the turkey at our mother's instruction. We stuffed the bird with the vegetable-bread mixed stuffing made beforehand, rubbed it with various seasonings. Thinking back, I'm surprised my mother allowed me to touch a raw turkey, even after washing my hands. In family photos, I'm reaching over the dinner table, with the netted tubing as my shirt, protecting my central line – I was so used to it by that point, I forgot it was there.

In almost all of my family photos dated to this period of recovery, as I'm walking around the house, I rarely had a shirt on, only wearing the netted tubing which supported my central line – going shirtless was a habit I picked up from my father, to remain cool during Texas heat.

I don't remember how my first Christmas after the transplant went, however, and that's usually a holiday so prominent in my memory. And while I don't remember sitting down to eat the turkey I helped prepare the next day, it's the day before Thanksgiving I remember fondly enough.

* * *

Every morning, I woke up and had to pester my mother into administrating Prograf and Bactrim to me, medication which suppressed my body's complete rejection of the transplant. They were gross and made me gag but I choked them down every morning – it was for my own good, I knew. And I was always diligent in remembering to take my meds.

However, as the months progressed, my dosage decreased, and at some point about eight months, I was told that I no longer had to take the Prograf medication and Bactrim at one year transplant anniversary. It came as a bit of a shock to me, as I believed that this was a procedure I had to get used to for life, as far as I was concerned. But it was a matter I only had to attend to for ten months, not ten years. And there was this odd sense of sadness I felt when I had to part from taking my meds, of course, I quickly got over it.

* * *

Despite my no longer having to stay at the hospital, I still had to return multiple times so that my health could be monitored for abnormalities in my recovery. It was bittersweet returning to Methodist Transplant Clinic, as I did get to reunite with some of the nurses who took care of me during my stay, yet I didn't want to be reminded of being cooped up in my room, separate from the life I was missing.

I never stayed overnight, thankfully, as it was usually just checking my labs, weight, blood pressure, blood, nutrition, among other vitals. As well as asking me how I felt after my transplant. I also turned in a chart my mother made me fill in upon my arrival home – it detailed what I ate, drunk and when, as well as the time and look of when I went to the bathroom; the color of my urine and poop. I'm assuming that gave the doctors a primary source as to how my body was reacting in its functions after the procedure.

Visits were several within a week, and it remained that way until about a month after I was released, where the doctors stated they didn't have to see me that often within the week, maybe two days a week instead of three, and now one day a week. Soon, I didn't have to be seen every week, it could be every other week. The waits between visits began to stretch out, with the doctors growing more and more confident and happy that I was responding satisfactory enough (besides a rash on my arms that soon went away) to be let out of their care. By the time third grade rolled around, I only had to see them monthly, and by the time fourth grade came, it was established that I would see them bi-yearly.

The nurses told me they didn't want to see me at the hospital again, after one of my visits, and I knew they meant it endearingly, in that they didn't want my health to regress and land me back into my suffocating room. I didn't want to be back either, and I responded well enough for that to come into reality.

* * *

Despite my not being able to return to school, my parents were determined that I still got some sort of education. The one I did get at the hospital was scarce, yet the one I got when I returned home was much better in my opinion. Ms. McCaskill reprised her role as my teacher and would come to my house on a weekly basis, bringing with her study sheets and DVDs ranging from math, English, and science.

One such day, as if it were a craft done in the classroom, we hid in my office as she gave me supplies to make a Mother's Day gift for my mother; I believe it was a small picture frame of me holding a sign of an exclamation of affection, but I can't remember clearly.

One time she brought a couple of The Magic School Bus discs, giving me my dose of science. And on another day, she dropped off a disc on Martin Luther King Jr. to watch – as if it were what she would put on for her own class – however, I hesitated to watch it at first, as I, for some reason, convinced myself I would see Mr. King get shot, and I was terrified. Of course, the film was only one summarizing his life's work, I found out as I eventually came to watch it.

On my birthday, Ms. McCaskill arrived with a cookie cake, McDonald's, and a purple tiara which she placed on my head. She celebrated my eighth birthday as a valuable member of the family.

I still continued my violin lessons as well, my parents wouldn't let me out of that too easily, either.

* * *

During one of my hospital visits, the doctors informed me that I was in a stable enough condition to step outside. Of course, I had to wear a hat and mask to prevent infection from bacteria, as well as keep from over-exposure to sun rays. I couldn't stay out for too long, nor could I roll in the grass or poke dead frogs I found – but I could step out and feel the wind my window had shielded me from for so long.

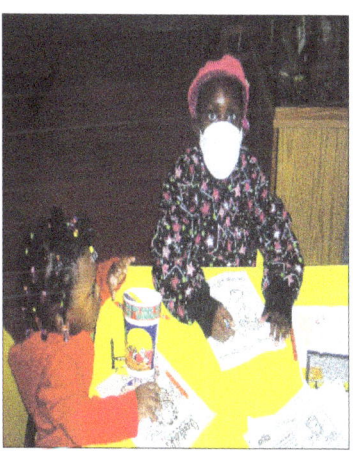

I couldn't even smell the air when I got to step out again, but I didn't mind the mask and hat hindrance – I was just happy I could be outside of my room again. It was so refreshing and I soaked up as much sun I could whenever I was permitted out.

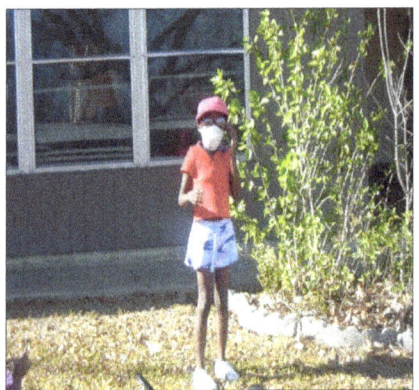 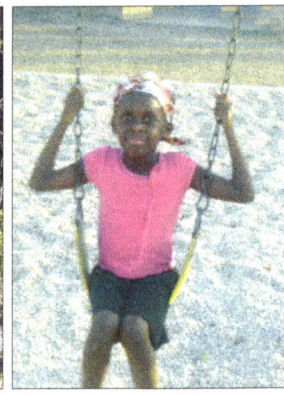

I was rid of the mask before I stopped wearing hats – my hair had grown back eventually, not to its formal length but enough to where I wasn't bald. But I liked the hats so I kept them in my wardrobe. But after several months, I didn't have to walk outside with a mask, and the taste of the air without the suffocating warmth of my own breath was heavenly.

By the time third grade began, I was permitted to return to school, amongst my peers, several of whom knew my story and were surprised to see me back in class, bombarding me with questions I was happy to answer.

* * *

I lost track of time – I don't remember seeing a calendar I could tick off, actually, I had gotten used to daily life in my sanitized bubble. I didn't complain of being almost isolated from the outside, of having to wear masks and hats when I did get to go outside, of my only destination apart from my home being Methodist, of having to choke down vile medication on the daily, of not being able to reunite with my school friends, of watching Mark and Aliah run about outside while all I could do was watch from my window, with the sanitized television as my only companion who I could get close to without fear of getting contaminated. This was all for my own good, after all. But as painful and excruciatingly long the wait was, it paid off in the end.

Goodbye, My Second Skin

Part of a home video I watched showed the general mood the night before I was getting my central line removed (Aliah was in the living room, watching TV and running towards my father upon his beckoning. She tripped and fell on a pillow, crying loudly after impact. Mark and I adore this part – we replayed it a number of times to Aliah's mortification). My mother was cleaning and replacing the dressing for the last time, while explaining to me that I would have to say goodbye to my port within the next twenty-four hours. I seemed happy, jovially thanking my parents for taking such good care of me, and slinging an arm around a dazed-looking Mark while thanking him as well. I don't remember feeling any apprehension until the next day.

My parents took Mark, Aliah, and I to Wilfred Hall Medical Center, San Antonio, Texas – another one of my secondary homes – where the removal was to take place, as did the insertion. I had my weight checked by an amiable nurse who also stayed with Mark while he waited for the procedure to be finished. We were then moved to a different room a few doors away. I was getting my blood pressure checked, a few doctors were coming in to brief my parents on the procedure, and this was when I started to feel scared.

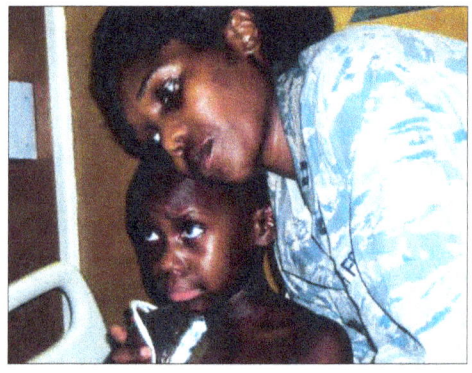

I do not remember what triggered the floodgates, but I began to cry at the thought of being separated from my central line. It had become a part of me – my skin had phased with the plastic tubing, grown around where it protruded as if it had always been there. I was so used to it – to feeling this inconsistent lump under my shirt, pressed against my skin. It was the mark of the beginning of my incredible journey, and its removal was the end, or rather, a huge step in reaching the end – an end which I did not know when I would reach.

And I of course did not picture the latter, more abstract thoughts as the reason of why I was afraid to part with my central line. I think, overall, I was terrified at the thought of them yanking it out of me, and my parents and the doctors reassured me that it would not be the case. I would definitely be put under and I wouldn't feel a thing.

There is a moment before the procedure happened that I will cherish forever, one which makes me acknowledge my mother's love, not to mention thank her a million times over for her support. She held me while I was crying and didn't let go even after I ceased crying. There is a nice photo of us on my Caringbridge website of us right before she carried me into the procedure room herself, no more tears or fears. I was ready to let go.

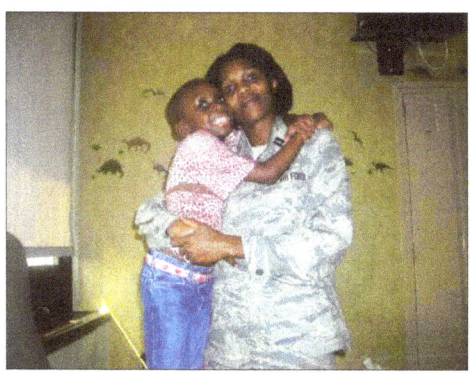

I expected to be put under and taken to the operation unit as I had months earlier, instead I was brought to a room across the hall from where Mark was waiting, surrounded by toys and TV. What stood out to me the most about the room was the black and white checkered tiled floors it had – I rarely saw that in real life and it was such a cartoonish concept to me, even as a kid. There were stickers of various characters from Disney Pixar's Cars, but I didn't catch that until I watched the home video. My father recorded the whole procedure, from taking my vitals, to my breakdown, to the tube being extracted.

I don't remember much of this part, only that I was given medication which was one step below knocking me out – my eyes were still open, apparently, but I have no recollection of the majority of the procedure. And I remember feeling no pain.

I remember coming to and being very disorientated, and clumsily tried to sit up, but the doctors kept gently pushing me back down. Once the room had stopped spinning about, Mark came into view, and I was eager to see him, though noted of the plethora of noses, mouths, and eyes he had, along with everyone else in the room. When we were cleared to leave, I remember attempting to walk by myself down the hall, but I fell, still very much uncoordinated, and my father carried me the rest of the way to the car.

When I managed to fully come to later on, my mother presented me with my second skin in a Ziploc bag. It was outside of me, fully, and the sight gave me a shiver. It still does, whenever I look at it. I was so used to looking down and seeing it right there. All I have left of its presence is a fading scar above the right side of my chest.

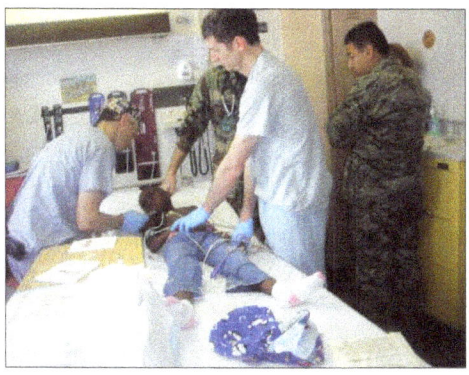

And it's funny, a few days after its removal I was rather morose, missing – oddly enough – and I felt the ghost of bundled tubes pressed against my chest. But I got over it quickly, and went on with my life. I was no longer restricted in movement, could bathe carefree, could forget about daily cleaning – I could finally let go.

Hello, Mr. President

This is the part of my story which perks just as many, if not more, ears than the transplant itself. Sometime before the summer of 2010, we received visitors. They were two representatives from the North Texas branch of the Make-A-Wish foundation, dedicated to granting the wishes of ailing children.

I was no longer an ailing child, but I still got whatever I wanted granted. I do not remember much of their visit, other than the fact that they sat me down in the living room, my parents a few feet away, and asked me: "Carol, what do you wish for?"

"I wish to meet the president."

Not the ordinary wish to visit Disneyland, but it was a wish nonetheless. The representatives gave me a little worksheet, where I drew the pillars of the White House for some reason I cannot remember. And then they left and I didn't hear back until the summer of 2010.

In the summer of 2010, my mother was deployed to Andrews Air Force Base in Maryland, and had been for quite some time. We had visited her a few months back for about a week – and an enjoyable one at that. Mark and I were in summer school and upon our return one day, my father told me that it was time for my wish to come true.

I had forgotten all about my wish to see the president, and it took some reminding from my father before I reached far enough in my memory to recall the meeting with the representatives. What a wonderful summer this would turn out to be.

We planned to meet my mother at hotel in Washington DC, and drive to wherever the hotel was. It was the Grand Hyatt, as grand as its name said, adorned with a colorful fountain situated in the center lobby which was the only thing I really recall about the hotel's structure.

After a missed flight and overnight stay at the airport, my family and I finally touched down in DC, whisked away to the hotel in what would be my first limo ride. We were a day behind schedule and had to scramble to prepare for meeting the president that day, with no room to breathe. I don't remember all of what happened when we arrived at the hotel, as well as the drive to the White House, but I can recall the visit to the point where I can write a solid chapter on my Executive Encounter.

We were walked around the White House halls – I can't remember most of them, they were probably adorned with antique paintings, ornate designs, as such. I remember standing by a large door, a bit agitated and wondering why we were waiting by a closed door, until it opened, and President Obama himself stepped out, beaming, looking down at this petite, slightly star-struck girl.

"Hi, Carol!" He greeted, one of the few things I remember him saying. I don't remember much of what myself or my family said, but he ushered us into his Oval Office. It was a bit smaller than I had envisioned, or perhaps that's just faded memory poking in holes. I don't remember many details about the Oval Office, I was wholly fixated on Mr. President.

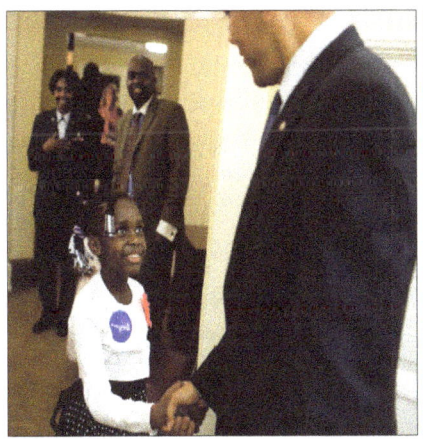
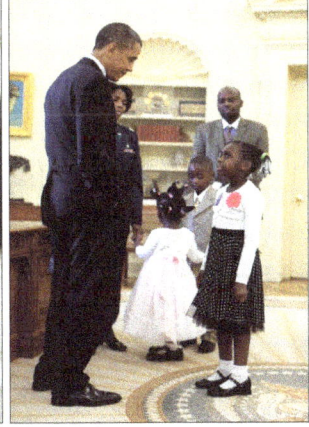

He spoke to my parents, asking where they were from, and exclaiming that we were basically related when they had answered with Uganda – Africans tend to claim anyone from Africa as their family, a show of light endearment, comradery. President Obama gave my brother a fist-bump which my mother still finds so amusing to this day and I don't remember if he interacted with Aliah.

My own interactions were somewhat rehearsed on my part, planned to near perfection beforehand. I had brought my violin to play for the President as a part of my presentation I had created. I had written and memorized a speech, and wow him with my decent violin skills. But security believed that I could have tucked a sinister surprise for the Commander-in-Chief in my violin case, so it was confiscated and I didn't get it back until the end of my visit. Of course, while I understand that security was their goal above all, I find it comical to imagine how a nine-year-old could harm such a tall man.

Despite this little hiccup in my planned presentation, my speech perfectly did the job meant for two. And by the end of it, President Obama was smiling in appreciation for my little rehearsed delivery. I don't remember what he said in response, but it was most likely along the lines of "I'll see what I can do" or something about acknowledging his role which I pointed out in my speech regarding helping kids affected by sickle cell. He gave me a blue bag which held a

Frisbee, yo-yo, two boxes of M&Ms, and a couple of pictures of his daughters' dog Bo. I still have the gifts to this day, and the M&Ms have never been opened.

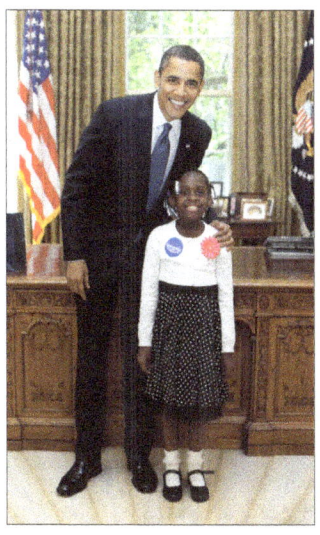

We took photos, made more small talk, and then he asked me if I would like to watch him take off in his Marine One helicopter. Normally, I asked my mother for permission before doing just about anything – but in that moment, I made the decision for myself (an enthusiastic "Yes") and then looked at her for approval afterwards.

We were led out of the Oval Office and outside to a field where the presidential helicopter was waiting for its very important passenger – there was already a crowd gathered to view its taking off, but my family and I were placed in the front, in prime viewing for all of the action. President Obama walked onto the field, waved, climbed in, and the helicopter took off. I distinctly remember the way the grass waved to and fro, resembling choppy sea water. I hadn't seen such movement before and that amused me more so than the helicopter taking off – but only for a moment. I turned my head up to see it lifting up and up, blades beating at the air with a deafening ferocity. My mother told me to hold down my dress to prevent the skirt from flying up, and every spectator's hand went to their eyes as flying particles made themselves known.

Once President Obama had made his exit, we started our tour of the White House, and the only rooms I can remember are the library, as well as the red, blue, and yellow rooms – mainly for their being named right after primary colors. My memory remains spotty for the rest of the day at the White House, but I fondly remember my family being whisked away to a restaurant afterwards, where I tried a steak good enough that it has remained seared in my memory. I didn't finish it though.

Make-A-Wish also planned a night tour about DC for my family and I, where we visited an aquarium (I got to pet a baby alligator whose tail had been injured by another alligator and got to take home a couple of dead shark eggs as a memento); took a tour on a trolley; visited the NationalMall (where I dropped a good portion of a hotdog I was enjoying on our way back from the Jefferson Memorial); and went on a guided tour of the Pentagon (our tour guide was a marine who walked backwards the whole time).

I flew home delighted, eager to tell my friends and teachers of the extraordinary trip I had, as well as attempt to finish the White House LEGO set I got and subsequently lost.

Chore List

Due to my always being a sickly child, my parents traded shifts in watching me and my siblings, or hired babysitters so that they could leave for work. It was a huge blessing when my grandmothers came to visit and care for us kids, taking a huge load off of my parents' plate.

My mother's mom, Grandma Deborah Namuddu, visited from Uganda at every child's birth, staying for a couple of months to help bathe, feed, and care for the newborn as well as watch the other kids. While I have few memories with my grandmother, my mother tells me she was a hard-working woman, coming from a humble background, Sesse Islands, in Uganda. She sacrificed to care for her family, building a substantial future for her kids, and my mother definitely took after her when she left for America.

It was in America that she met my other grandmother – Grandma Carol. A kindly woman who took her in as her own daughter, raising her as she found her footing on new soil. I was named after Grandma Carol, and I can remember her visits on Mark and Aliah's birth, as well as many others in between.

My illness and recovery stunted what time my parents could have used to train me in household chores, as well as prohibit me from caring for my siblings. When I started regaining my strength after the procedure, and was well enough to take on more physical exertion, my parents slowly taught me simple household chores, and how to cook simple meals. I memorized their cellphone and work phone numbers, to use in case of an emergency.

One such emergency that happened while I was babysitting my siblings, and the summer heat made me crave soup. I ended up boiling onions and tomatoes, thinking it would turn the water into broth, and after stirring vigorously, the water splashed onto my shirt. I later found out I had gotten a small burn on my stomach – it scarred and leaves me with a story I love to recount.

Besides acting as a little caretaker, I had to step up my role as sort of a surrogate parent towards my siblings, in aiding with their homework, getting them dressed and ready for school, feeding them, and the like. I was a kid myself, but I began acting like a smaller adult, herding instead of playing with Mark and Aliah, concerned if they had eaten that day or were prepared for the next day, rather than concerning myself on what game we would all play. As I got older and I had gained the trust of my parents, they were both able to leave the house to work, while I took care of the house.

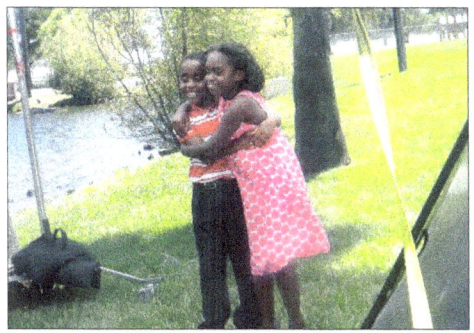

The shift I had made from a child who mainly stayed bedridden to a child who ran the house like clockwork was, least to say, extreme, almost with a whiplash effect when I think about it. I find it peculiar, even humorous that I slingshot from a helpless child to one who could help herself as well as the rest of her family. Of course, I think this newfound stepping ground gave me the ability to move forward in utilizing my experiences to my benefit, as well as to the benefit of others.

Growing up in a military family as the eldest child, I automatically assumed the role of a parent when the time came for me to step up. When I was thirteen, my mother deployed to Afghanistan, and my father worked night shift. As such, it was time for me to act as the surrogate parent to my brother and sister.

My siblings were still in elementary school, and they needed help for checking over their work, picking out their clothes, reminders of when it was time to leave for the bus – tasks which parents usually fill, but not in our case. I answered every homework problem, woke them up for school, herded them out before the bus left, did just about everything a parent does for getting their kid prepared for school.

Of course, it wasn't easy. I wasn't a parent, I had work to do, too, and as overwhelming as it was at times, the dynamics had changed. With my parents out of the picture most of the time, I began to run the house like clockwork. And that dynamic has persisted even today. Even though now my parents are home, my siblings almost always go to me first for just about anything, and my parents second.

And this parenting role extends beyond my family. In 2018, I signed up as a Link Leader in a new program my school implemented, where upperclassmen guide new students throughout high school. I was given a group of eight kids and invited them to orientation, conducted ice breaker games, passed out schedules, and guided them about the campus.

Link Leadership is something which was entirely out of my comfort zone, but I am at least confident that by now, the kids I've mentored have found their way about the school and settled into their first year in high school smoothly. After all, they had the helping hand that I didn't have my first year. I continued to be their resource and they have my number and I encourage them to reach me at any time.

Grandma Carol

I am the namesake of a modest woman who has lived in the Northeastern part of America for most of her life. All of my memories of her are nothing but warm, comfortable, enriching, and loving. She was a woman who dedicated her entire life to her faith and aiding others in the name of her beliefs, indulging on the success of others with her helping hand, rather than gluttonous pleasures of TV, vacations, and expensive items.

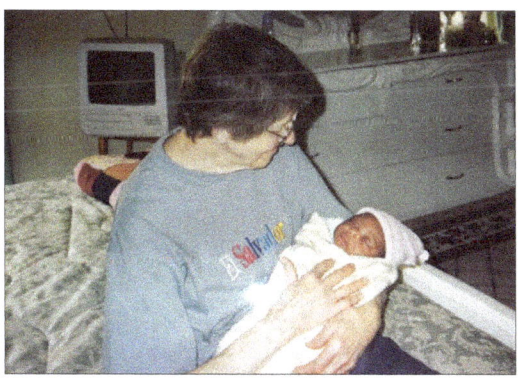

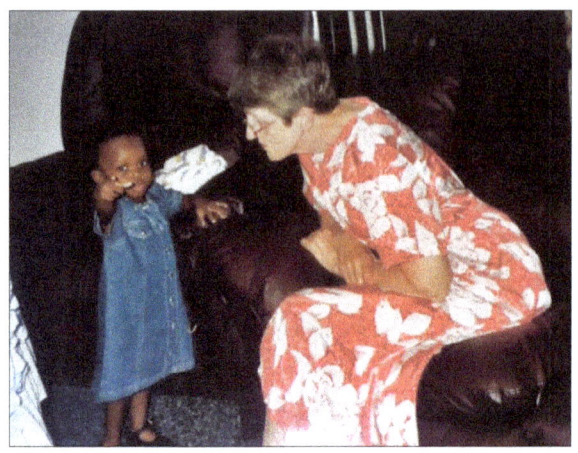

She was polite, always smiling, and incredibly intelligent. She was quiet, yet when she spoke, her words were never without impact. I often found her diving intently into her latest read, pushing her glasses up to inform me all about what she had in her hands.

Grandma Carol LeClaire always wanted to have a family, but the direction which her faithful life had run made it seemingly impossible for her goal to be reached. Until my mother, fresh from Africa with no one to turn to landed on American soil. A priest named Father Mark (my brother is his namesake as well) heard of my mother's predicament, her need to stay somewhere warm and comforting and safe for her start in America – and so he brought her to Grandma Carol.

My mother got a loving home to lay her roots down in America and Grandma Carol got the daughter she had always wanted. My mother fondly recalls their domestic life together, where they would eat breakfast together, walk to the nearby store to run errands, live together as if they were mother and daughter.

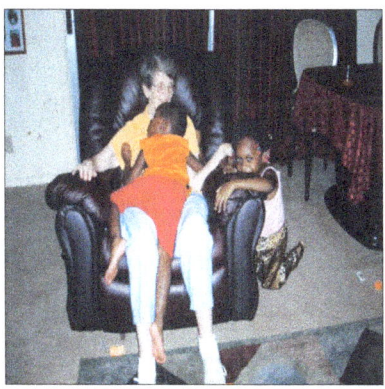

Grandma Carol introduced my mother to her own family as well, people such as her younger brother Uncle Don would come to welcome my mother and recognize her as Grandma's daughter. Still smiling fondly in reminiscing of how much she loved my mother.

Grandma Carol supported my mother all throughout her college career, proudly standing by her at graduation as she received her Nursing degree hugging her daughter tightly with a loving "You did it!" Grandma's support lay the groundwork for my mother in hitting the pavement with extraordinary force, reaching above the baseline requirements.

Grandma Carol proudly held her sick namesake hours after she was born, glowing with absolute joy when she answered to the name of Carol once her ears developed.

She had a picture of her, willingly gushing about her granddaughter should anyone have asked.

Grandma Carol held, sang to, read to, and nurtured three grandchildren, all of whom crowded around her coveted rocking chair upon her visits, drinking in whatever story she told them.

I fondly remember Grandma Carol reading Alice in Wonderland to me; and helping me practice for the spelling bee competition; and sending me a doll she made out of cloth and shoelaces herself named Sally, who still holds a place of honor on my headboard; and staying up for hours with me engaged in conversation on just about any topic, no matter how old I was. Grandma Carol would hold me on a swing chair, sang for me as I battled pain due to sickle cell. She also sent out letters to several religious places asking for prayers during my transplant journey. These memories are all I have left of her, as she passed away on February 27th, in 2018. I didn't weep as much as I thought I would, for I knew that in the end, Grandma Carol felt she had lived a satisfactory, and fruitful life, bearing a family which she had always wanted, who still miss her very much. I absolutely love and cherish my Grandma Carol, and it would be criminal not to write a dedication in her honor. After all, I credit her with much of the good fortune I have now.

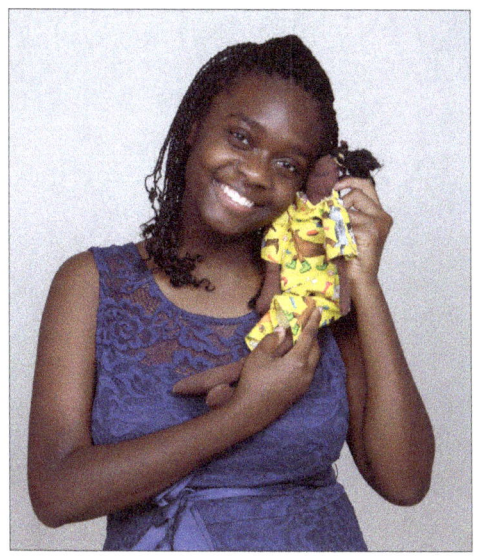

Sally (doll) a valuable gift from grandma

Alternative Path

The only way to get awareness out there is to keep running your mouth, was basically along the lines of what my mother says about Sickle Cell. The issue of lack of sufficient healthcare in Uganda – especially for Sickle Cell patients – still was prevalent, and the only way for the issue to gain attention is to keep flapping your lips, getting as many ears to listen.

It wasn't until sometime after my return to school that I started telling my transplant story to local news channels. There was one affiliated with Lackland Air Force in Texas, which I briefly spoke to – the interview made me miss the first half of school and I ate lunch late that day.

In 2010, my family and I flew to Uganda where they held a Sickle Cell Conference for the then Ugandan American Sickle Cell Rescue Fund they had started back around my diagnosis. Before that, however, there was walk to raise awareness, and I proudly remember completing the whole length, even after my parents had asked multiple times if I wished to stop for a break.

During the Conference, I sat up on stage with my parents as they talked in their native tongue to the crowd about what I didn't know. But what I was to do was rehearsed, I would say "My name is Carol Marriam Mulumba, and I am going to play my violin for you" and I performed a few songs as a microphone was dangled above my instrument. Then I introduced a then popular Ugandan singer Eddie Kenzo who further entertained those in attendance. I later helped my mother pass out gifts and cake, and then I went home.

At the time, I didn't understand why I had to be there – I never gave it much thought, really – but I now know that I was there to quietly say to those affiliated with Sickle Cell that there was hope, and I was proof of that.

In 2010, due to military orders, my family had to pack up and leave behind all of the amazing people we met in Texas, and move to Travis Air Force Base, California. I tried stalling the move by insisting that California had water issues, and therefore wouldn't be the most ideal place to live – that didn't change military orders, and we soon called Travis Air Force Base home. Adjusting took time, but I eventually found a comfortable niche in California. In addition, I was to still be seen at a children's hospital in Oakland, just to monitor my health status after the transplant.

After moving to California, in 2010, I spoke about my Sickle Cell story at the Cord Blood Registry (CBR), San Bruno in San Francisco, showing the relative success of the Bone Marrow Transplant and Cord Blood for the treatment of Sickle Cell. My parents also thanked CBR for saving Mark and Aliah's cord blood for free.

In 2015, right after I finished eighth grade, we flew back to Uganda for another conference, where I became much more active. I accompanied my mother to various TV appearances and mini conferences, briefly talking about my experience and encouraging viewers to attend the Sickle Cell Conference. There was a radio broadcast which my mother and I attended where, despite my being terribly ill from stomach flu, I managed to choke out of my aspirations for the future of health care in Uganda – take away the stigma and replace it with a structure of universal care for all, regardless of ailments and backgrounds.

There was a larger crowd at my second conference than my first, and I was able to better articulate myself as a fourteen year old than a nine year old. I had a PowerPoint prepared with an accompanying speech, walking the audience through my life, from diagnosis, to multiple nights of pain and despair, to the transplant, its arduous recovery, up to the present. Every now and then I'd glance into the crowd – I was taught to always look at the crowd during a speech – and I saw many glassy eyes and running tears. Even my mother was crying, I saw, as I glanced at her.

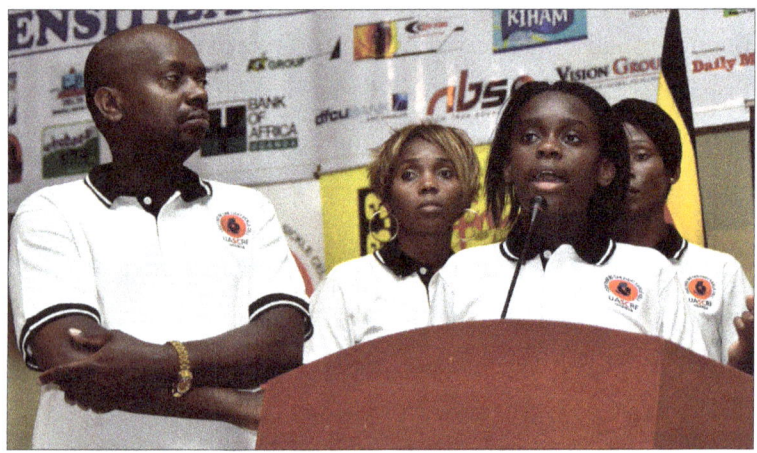

4th Sickle Cell Conference, Kampala, Uganda

I was shaking yet finished strong, and after my speech, my father translated everything in the local language, Luganda – I got a stronger applause once everyone could understand all that I was saying.

I haven't been to Uganda since 2015, but I haven't stopped speaking about Sickle Cell. This book is such an example. Of course, besides speaking out, I have also been pursuing my goal of higher education. I've recently graduated from Vanden High school and come this fall, I will be entering, not a casket, but a college. I plan on studying biology at the University of California in Los Angeles so that I may be one step closer to becoming a doctor, aiding children who are as unfortunate as I was, struck with an unlucky arrow in their genetic code.

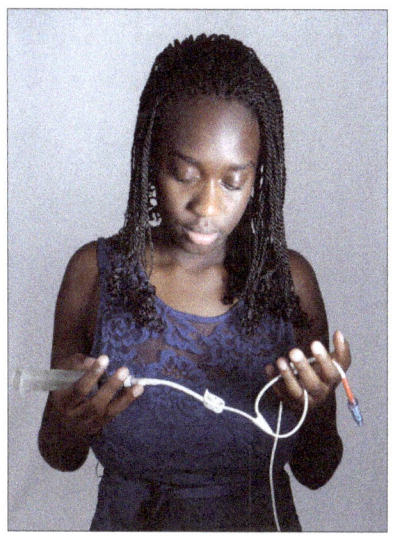

It was once part of "skin"

Of course, I have a long way to go before I gain the title of Doctor and can get to work on treating patients, but I always find it a little humorous that eighteen years ago I was doomed to die within the next few years, yet I was flung in a totally different direction ten years ago. We celebrate October 29th (bone marrow) and 31st (cord blood) transplant every year as a second birthday for me, the day I sidestepped my intended fate for a path much more fruitful and fulfilling. A path where my life wouldn't be cut short, where I would walk amongst my peers on ground which I couldn't reach as a child, but could finally step up to now that I'm grown. I was given a future dedicated to healing others, as I have been healed.

I'd like to go back in time to reassure little Carol that the casket wouldn't be getting to me for a long while.

Acknowledgements

There are multiple people I must thank who have helped me throughout my life, such as the staff at Children's Hospital of Michigan, Wilford Hall Medical Center-Texas, Methodist Children's Hospital-Texas, Oakland Children's Hospital-California for treating me on my worst days, better days, and ensuring my ultimate recovery and making hospital stays bearable.

The Cord blood registry (CBR) for saving my brother Mark's cord blood for free.

The teachers and staff – especially the nurses office- at Lackland Elementary School-San Antonio, Texas for always being so understanding whenever I had to leave early, visit the nurse's office, hospital emergency room, or miss days on end.

Grandma Carol's family who I have come to know as my own.

Grandma Carol for caring for my mother upon her entry in America, and making her feel welcome and loved on new soil.

Grandma Deborah for instilling a fighting spirit within my mother which spurned her into reaching for high goals, such as a life in America.

My friends who I have met over the years, who never made me feel like I was different with my illness.

My family for their unwavering support since birth, and whose love I will fiercely cherish for life.

About the Author

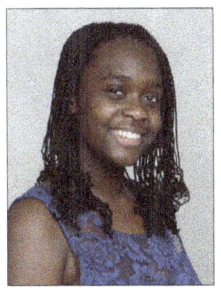

Carol Mulumba is a freshman at the University of California, Los Angeles (UCAL). Currently studying molecular biology, she aspires to become a medical doctor. She was featured in several news papers, televisions, and in the Be The Match Bone Marrow Transplant, Super Sam vs Marrow Monsters Pediatric video, "20-minute award-winning, animated film featuring Sam, a young boy making an epic movie production about his own transplant experience."

Contact: Mom's e-mail address: nlukiah@yahoo.com

www.ingramcontent.com/pod-product-compliance
Lightning Source LLC
Chambersburg PA
CBHW070303010526
44108CB00039B/1710